Drying My Tears

One Family's Journey with Autoimmunity

Liz Wilkey

Acknowledgements

Thank goodness for all the things you are not,
thank goodness you're not something someone forgot,
and left all alone in some punkerish place,
like a rusty tin coat hanger hanging in space.
— *Dr. Seuss*

My thanks go out to my husband, Michael, for his care for me and support for this memoir. I also want to express my gratitude to my three daughters and two brothers who have allowed their stories to be told.

Thanks also to my good friend, Jeanne Kappel; my fellow Sjogren's sufferer, Kate Stout; and my sister-in-law, Cate Harty for reading, editing, and encouraging me to record my story.

This story regarding my family's health challenges would not be complete without the excellent medical care given to us by Doctor Thomas Lehman, Chief of Pediatric Rheumatology at The Hospital for Special Surgery (New York) Doctor Julius Birnbuam of The Jerome L. Greene Sjogren's Syndrome Center at Johns Hopkins (Baltimore) and Doctor Shari Flowers of Skylands Medical Group in Randolph, N.J. You have all served as beacons of hope in the often-murky waters of autoimmunity. I feel compelled, however, to add a disclaimer that if any of the medical information or terminology I have included in this book is over-simplified or incorrect, it cannot be attributed to these excellent physicians, but to this author who then should – indeed – be sent to some punkerish place, like a rusty tin coat hanger hanging in space.

This book is dedicated to my three
beautiful, resilient, and determined daughters:
Kaitlyn, Megan, and Leah.

Foreword

From Virginia Ladd
President and Executive Director
American Autoimmune Related Diseases Association

Liz's story is all too common in the autoimmune disease community. More than 50 million Americans have been diagnosed with at least one autoimmune disease. As Liz's story demonstrates, autoimmune diseases run in families, not a single disease, like lupus or Hashimoto's, but the category of disease. By bringing awareness to this disease category, we hope that more people will know that it is an important part of a family's medical history.

A survey conducted by the American Autoimmune Diseases Association (AARDA) found that it takes on average three years and examinations by four doctors before someone receives an accurate autoimmune disease diagnosis. By becoming aware and knowing their family history, patients will know to ask about the autoimmune connection. Additionally, AARDA seeks to education health care professionals about symptoms and treatments to get patients quicker diagnoses and better care.

As Liz has personally experienced, autoimmune diseases not only cluster in families but also in people. Having multiple diseases is another commonality in the autoimmune community. To further understand this phenomenon and to help scientists and researchers study these connections,

AARDA developed the Autoimmune Research Network, or ARNet. This database gathers patient-powered data to connect the scientific and research communities to the patients; including opportunities for clinical trials which lead to breakthroughs throughout the autoimmune disease community.

We hope that patients find strength to speak up and speak out about autoimmune disease. Even more, we hope that patients are encouraged and gain hope from Liz's story. Laughter is the best medicine. Having a good sense of humor and a strong support system can make all the difference in living and thriving with these diseases.

Sincerely,

Virginia Ladd
President and Executive Director

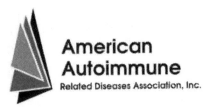

Preface

I have heard there are troubles of more than one kind,
some come from ahead, some come from behind.
But I've bought a big bat,
I'm all ready you see;
now my troubles are going to have troubles with me.

– Dr. Seuss

Troubles. I suppose that every one of us faces troubles of one kind or another. My own personal troubles revolve around a certain word which has an effect on upwards of 50 million Americans as well. That word? Autoimmunity. The following is just a primer of what my troubles have caused me to learn about a certain set of disorders which carry the label, "Autoimmune Diseases."

I know that there are between 80–100 serious, chronic illnesses in which autoimmunity is the underlying cause. These illnesses can involve almost every human organ system.

I have learned that these diseases, syndromes, and disorders have one thing in common: because of some mixed-up stimuli, the fighter cells in your body start to mistake healthy tissue for a virus or intruder and begin to attack the very organs they were designed to protect.

I understand that a tendency to develop autoimmune diseases is thought to be inherited. This predisposition may be large or small depending on the disease but, in general, close relatives are more likely to develop the same or a related autoimmune disease.

I now know that this tendency alone is not the determining factor in whether or not any one individual develops an autoimmune disease. It is likely that environmental factors acting along with genetic predisposition are responsible for triggering the onset of disease.

I can now tell you with certainty that those with the greatest risk of developing an autoimmune disease are those who have already been diagnosed with another.

I have learned that most people who battle with autoimmune diseases also suffer from fatigue, malaise, joint and muscle pain, fever, and a general sense of feeling unwell. Many of these diseases are referred to as "invisible illnesses" because those who suffer from them often do not look sick on the outside.

I know that there is no cure for autoimmune diseases and treatment is most often aimed at halting or slowing the progression of these conditions. In some cases, treatment is only aimed at relieving the discomfort of various symptoms.

I now know that, although estimates vary widely, there are between 23 and 50 million Americans living and coping with autoimmune diseases.

I recognize the fact that I am one of them myself and directly related to five others.

Yet simply knowing about my troubles is not enough for me. I believe it is time that others become educated about these diseases as well. If up to 50 million Americans are suffering from autoimmune-related conditions, why is it we hear so little about them? Is it because they are often strange sounding and unpronounceable, like Sjogren's Syndrome, Guillain-Barre, Scleroderma, or Hashimoto's Thyroiditis? Is it due to the fact that they are, indeed, invisible illnesses? That they are not lumped together in one big, scary word like "cancer?"

My hope is that by reading my story you will not only learn about the particular diseases which have affected my family, but will gain insight into what it feels like to live with chronic illness. I will not bombard you with in-depth medical information, but only offer you a certain level of awareness. I want to show you the path to being a better spouse, sibling, child, or friend of someone who suffers from autoimmunity.

And if you, like me, are the one who battles with an autoimmune disease, I hope that relating my personal journey will help to lessen the feelings of isolation which often arise when others are misinformed or not attentive to our plight. I also want to share my experiences of integrating complementary methods of healing with traditional medical approaches and offer you ideas for developing a mindset which will allow you to absorb all of the healing energies available to you.

I beg you not to judge me flippant, glib, or dismissive as I relate my symptoms or those of my daughters in the upcoming pages. I trust that you will recognize humor for the cathartic release which it serves here. I invite you to laugh along and let your own tears become mine when I attempt to cry. I dare hope you even find yourself fighting the urge to bite your fingernails a time or two. If so, I have done my job and you will have gained a perspective on what it is like to live in the world of autoimmunity.

After all, even though I thought I had learned how to navigate the storm watching my own children suffer with different autoimmune processes, it wasn't until I had to steer through the tumult of my own personal tempest that I knew more than facts. I quickly learned that I needed to do something to, indeed, give my troubles, troubles with me!

Introduction

Today I shall behave as if this is the day I will be remembered.
– Dr. Seuss

Did you ever wake up one morning thinking your life should be displayed on the big screen? Have you thought about what it would look like? How the opening scenes would play out? What the soundtrack verifying your very existence would be?

I attended a screening of a movie the other day. I know that some of you may now be wondering why a certified mouse-a-phobic would forsake her ban on stepping into a sticky-floored-popcorn-strewn-rodent-paradise simply to watch a film which would be available for home viewing in a few short months. The answer lies with the newly renovated theater outfitted with reclining seats which, through accident of design, now protect me from my phobia of an errant rodent running over my feet while I'm engrossed in my movie viewing.

Given that the movie I happened to be engrossed in was based on the true story of a woman who did nothing more than invent a mere mop, I now know that any story – including my own – can be made to be equally compelling. And so I have determined that the opening scene of my movie would look like this:

Woman in a white spa bathrobe slides past a Tibetan
singing bowl, emerges from a misty, ethereal, Zen-inspired

bedroom and tiptoes somewhat gingerly down the stairs of her home early in the morning. (Call it a pain-filled hobble in the screenplay if you must.) Stifling her morning cough, it is clear that she is trying not to wake others in her household so that she can spend these pre-dawn moments to herself.

She is greeted by the light-pawed steps of Giardia Jax. Not that the cat's name was ever meant to indicate an intestinal outrage, it simply became one of those nicknames that happened to stick because of the unfortunate parasite which has plagued the poor tabby since the day he was adopted just four short months ago. Next on the scene appears Kasey, the woman's 11-year-old retriever, whose name is not preceded by any disease because that sweetheart of a dog has never carried anything more than an occasional tick into this frenzied household.

The woman smiles to herself thinking – just thinking – what it would be like if every member of her family were to wear their eponymous and funny-sounding diseases along with their names. Why are these illnesses she deals with so strange sounding? Has there never been a doctor with a simple last name who gave their name to a disease they've identified? But have no fear; our leading lady loves the thought of the fanciful and absurd.

And she loves alliteration.

She whispers these thoughts to Kasey. Since she is named Liz, perhaps she should be the one in the household who suffers most from lupus, yet she could never turn around and wish her own alliterative disease on one of her daughters. Besides, she doesn't have a daughter named Suzie or Sara. She supposes that she and her husband should have named those three girls differently. With the host of autoimmune diseases which now live in her house, *all sorts of names would have worked. And who knows, the way things continue to unfold in her life, the list may yet be extended.*

Back now to the dog.

It is clear that Kasey knows the drill. Although this particular human has not been the first one downstairs in many a day, the sleeping patterns of the woman who runs this house are so erratic that the dog has long abandoned all sense of routine. She also knows that she must remain silent when the woman whispers all those lovely things to her in the wee hours of the morning. Above all, the dog is quite positive that whichever human springs her from her crate will make sure that the morning manna will very shortly be dropping from heaven in the form of some kibble in her food bowl.

But as the woman is dishing the food into the respective animal's bowls, the toilet flushes in the room overhead and it becomes evident to all who hear it that the dog is the only one in the scene who is going to get a taste of heaven on this particular morning.

And then the opening credits start rolling.

But perhaps the opening scene would be more effective if it were that which had transpired two minutes earlier in our heroine's bedroom:

A woman, after tussling with a snow-white comforter, flings the accursed quilt off of her single bed and blindly gropes for a vial of eye drops from a windowsill littered with sprays, ointments, and pill bottles. After dispensing a drop into each of her eyes, she gulps down the first of her morning medications, shuts off the bothersome spray of her misting room humidifier, rips the wrapping from her wrist splints, and cries aloud to God above, "This life which you have given me is becoming unbearable!" The accompanying sobbing is unusual in several ways – not only is it silent, it is tearless. It is also unique in that it betrays the depths of a genie which she rarely lets out of its bottle; for after all, our leading lady's despair is as deep and as hollow as the gong that is emitted from that singing bowl.

And now please roll the opening credits.

But wait movie viewers, we have one more choice. Perhaps the film should have started rolling just a few seconds before the preceding scene like the true horror film it represents:

Our protagonist awakes screaming from a nightmare in which she is being eaten by ants. Struggling to rid herself of thousands of ravenous pincers, she wrestles to liberate her body from a tangle of bedclothes, reflexively connecting them to her dream. Once freed and half-awake, she immediately knows that this nightmare – like so many preceding ones – was grounded in reality, for she recognizes the all-too-familiar sensation of what she can only describe as a morning "skin ache."

When I begin to use terms like "protagonist" in place of "leading lady" I know my story belongs in written form; for which actress would they choose to portray me? Casting directors would be forced to redesign me, transforming my character to someone graceful and petite because no one likes to watch an overweight woman in her fifties for two long hours. No matter how much they would try to ugly her down as she glances in the mirror upon awakening, no living soul can look quite as imperfect as I do while wiping away the crust the nighttime eye drops have left on my lashes and lids. And, Oscar winner or not, that woman would never be able to replicate with any accuracy the way I stick my tongue out at my reflection once that army of gray hair has been spied making a flanking maneuver across my part line just three weeks after having beaten them into retreat at the beauty salon. Those actresses continue to look beautiful even when the hair and make-up artists are convinced they have made them out to be sad, or wistful, or tired, or depressed, or sickly – all of which they would have to be if they wanted to play the role of me.

But whichever, memoirs or movie, my story would continue:

Our heroine then proceeds to tiptoe through the kitchen and continue her morning ritual by brewing a pot of green tea and choosing her "Celtic Spa" playlist on her iPod. She opens the door to the refrigerator – rifling past health juices, blocks of cheese, medical injection pens, kitty cat probiotics, and her sizable box of wine – until she unearths the object of her hunt and proceeds to add precisely five drops of organic sweetener into the pot. The hopeful soul then attempts to absorb invisible energies by pouring the tea into her "healing touch" mug embedded with a crystal that promises the holder improved health and energy with every sip.

In an effort to deflect conversation with her husband (who we all suspect was the instigator of the toilet flush) she heats her moisturizing eye goggles, rearranges the myriad of pillows resting on the living room couch, and plops down on the corner where she has resided for the better part of the last two years. She then lights the candle in her Himalayan salt lamp, dons those goggles, and proceeds to play a private cameo role of contented blind woman petting her guide dog.

Our leading lady is simply not in the mood for morning conversation today. She wants silence. If her dentist had suggested an appliance to alleviate her dry mouth symptoms, she would have employed that with all alacrity if it ensured warding off attempts at dialogue. Its very existence would have complicated the tea drinking, but she could always take up her daughters' habit of using straws while consuming beverages like coffee, tea, and red wine in order to maintain their perfectly whitened teeth.

Turns out there was no need to have worried about employing prophylactic measures for conjugal conversation this morning, for after they each utter an obligatory, "Good morning," it becomes clear to her that the man of the house has other things on his mind as well. The coffee machine quickly brews two cups of decaf which he silently downs before she hears the treadmill revving up in the basement below. Aaaah, this is a running morning for him. She can't quite keep his fitness regime straight; one day is the same as the next in her life.

No need either this time to worry about which Hollywood actor will play the leading man if by chance her book becomes a film. The husband in this story has aged handsomely and the compelling worry over his own heart health has done the rest. Unlike his wife of 30 years, this man's morning mirror inspection smiles back at him.

A half-hour run, quick shower along with his kale protein drink, and he's out the door. No time for a goodbye kiss. No perceptive last-minute glance in search of the dried tracks of his wife's tears. That stuff is reserved for Hollywood; and for people whose bodies allow them to make tears. Although, if that husband had been bestowed with superhuman eyesight, he just may have spied the lone rivulet of one sweetly-savored drop that fell, not as a herald of others to come, but as the singular courier which her stingy disease had allowed her to wring out of an ocean of misery.

Yet, because she offered him no hint, none was received. This woman, although deficient in many areas, could confidently be called a Master of Disguise.

Once the garage door clamors shut, she brings the war-torn comforter down from her bedroom floor and settles once more onto her couch corner. It is clear that she still has things to accomplish before the two remaining occupants of the house arise. When push comes to shove, this tea-and-Buddha-loving-wannabe is a devout Christian fiercely in need of her prayer and meditation time this morning.

Try as she might to keep her mind focused, she finds her thoughts wandering back to her evening out the night before and knows that her own behavior is that which lies behind her morning disposition. The night only reaffirmed how far apart she has grown from others and fills her with a sense of shame and humiliation. She is ashamed of the undeniable envy she felt as she listened to others recount the details of a night out with those who had once been her own co-workers as well; horrified at one particular barb that seemed to leap from her lips uninvited; embarrassed that she can no longer make small talk and abhors it when others do; guilty for the little hash marks she lines up in her head for each hurt endured when those she encounters never ask after her family's health, for she thinks – no, is certain – that others are convinced that she has made the whole nightmare up; mortified, because she knows in her heart that God sees through her pretense of trying to act cheerful as she asks after the comings and goings of other's lives.

But all who have followed her story so far can sense that she was right in her early morning railings. The life she is leading has indeed grown intolerable. She inclines her head towards heaven and asks, "How on earth did it get to be like this? My children sick? My own life forever altered by unceasing illness? Walling myself off from my husband?

Becoming isolated from family and friends? And when, dear Lord, when will things get better? Please tell me when!"

Her eyes (and, perchance, the camera) then pan to the new toy Santa just happened to bring the dog a few short weeks ago: a pink pig with silver wings. Even our heroine is astute enough to know that THAT pig is never going to fly. This is the precise moment that she decides to abandon writing her manuscript of children's poetry and replace it with documenting the story of her family's illnesses. Above all, she vows that she will continue to write until her arthritic and tremor-ridden fingers fall off.

Even though film has now turned to print, we still need to add a soundtrack to my story, for I am a firm believer that there is a steady stream of music at play behind each of our lives. Although I have always pictured a Billie Holiday album as the backdrop to my life, you – for your own reading enjoyment – can feel free to choose from any of the playlists on my iPod. My preference would be that you browse within my new age, Celtic, and jazz files, but since I have two thousand songs on that little device you can consider my musical world your oyster. I do, however, have the following requirements:

Be sure to include my personal anthem, *Wonder* by Natalie Merchant and a song or two about various heartaches from Patsy Cline. *She's Come Undun* by The Guess Who is essential and, in truth, should be substituted for the title of this memoir. Future chapters will unveil the precise reasons why you need to include Coldplay's *Yellow* along with Joni Mitchell's *Both Sides Now,* and Jackson Browne's *Doctor My Eyes.*

I used to have a playlist tagged "Motherhood" filled with whimsical songs I loved to sing to my daughters in those blissful days when they were young – songs like *Part of Your World, Hakuna Matata,* and *Baby Mine.* I deleted that list a few years ago when it became clear that wishing on a star did not make my dreams come true. You, however, may want to resurrect these as I relate the tales of my daughters' childhood years in upcoming pages.

While viewing that movie the other day I was reminded of the sentiment which floods my very being every time I hear *Expecting to Fly* by Buffalo Springfield. The emotional genius behind that song is more than my poor heart can handle and finds me longing to display the same brilliance in my own writing. You can find this song in my "Psycho Sixties" list. Not that I have an overwhelming affinity for music of the Sixties, but I do possess an irresistible urge to tuck my music – and my life – into tidy lists.

But unless you love hyphens as much as I do, no single list, word, or label could ever capture the wine-gulping-cheese-consuming-mouse-fearing-punctuation-flinging-celtic-and-Buddha-loving paradox that is me.

So please allow me to return to our cinematic vista one more time.

The scene opens as our heroine sits with tea and laptop later that day. Reflecting on her story, a tale which she has blended and stirred so many times that it now seems to be steeped in sadness, she is reminded of that single poem which she forever holds in her heart. This lyrical wonder is infused with her beloved Irish melancholy and I beg you to savor its essence too. Feel free to read it aloud with her. Better yet, take the time to memorize it and recite it with quiet passion. When you do, you – too – will hear it in your deep heart's core.

When You Are Old

When you are old and grey and full of sleep
And nodding by the fire, take down this book,
And slowly read, and dream of the soft look
Your eyes had once, and of their shadows deep.

How many loved your moments of glad grace,
And loved your beauty with love false or true,
But one man loved the pilgrim soul in you,
And loved the sorrows of your changing face;

And bending down beside the glowing bars,
Murmur, a little sadly, how Love fled
And paced upon the mountains overhead
And hid his face amid a crowd of stars.

– *William Butler Yeats*

Rest assured, our leading lady's husband has not become a darting mountain man, nor is her life devoid of love, yet Yeats' arrow has hit its mark in countless other ways. And while – thanks to those trips to the beauty salon – the heroine of our story may not be gray for years to come, I believe that an errant few would have described her as having a certain sense of beauty in her younger days when she still possessed those "moments of glad grace." As the camera flashes back to a scene of her wedding day, our viewers are able to get a glimpse for themselves.

But this poem points to sorrow, to loss, to want. What is it that has fled? Innocence? Hope? A certitude that things will come right at the end? For our poor heroine knows that her pilgrim soul has wandered into uncharted territory a few too many times for her liking. What's more, she is quite sure that her shadowed eyes could no longer be called "soft." And *in truth, she is no longer certain she is capable of allowing anyone to love the sorrows of her changing face.*

I suppose it is time for you, my reader, to determine for yourself.

Part One: My Story

1. First Comes Love, then Comes. . .

We are all a little weird and life's a little weird,
and when we find someone whose weirdness is compatible with ours,
we join up with them and fall in mutual weirdness and call it love.
– Dr. Seuss

Marriage

It is perfectly safe to say that I married for my children.

It is a truth universally acknowledged that people marry for various reasons. Some happy couples jump into matrimony with wild abandon. Some see their friends and contemporaries marrying and feel their time has come too. Some tie the knot for security; others for companionship. Some, I venture to guess, get hitched simply for the party. And some people marry because of their desire to have children and start a family.

I was clearly one of the kid-craving kind.

It is not that I feared that a tattered biological clock was ticking away inside of me; I was a mere 27 at the time. And it is not that I wasn't ecstatically happy. I sincerely loved my husband-to-be with all my heart. Standing before the altar on that sunny day in late November, I eagerly awaited the big question – the one that would come before the "to have and to hold in sickness and health" part, for I knew that during the nuptials, we would state our intentions when the officiant asked:

Will you accept children lovingly from God, and bring them up according to the law of Christ and his Church?

My heart leapt for joy, waiting for the chance to declare:

Yes! Yes! And Yes!

The astute reader will note that there were only two questions yet I offered three responses, but that only represents my level of enthusiasm regarding becoming a mother. My wedding day was not about the reception, photographer, or bridesmaids' dresses; it was a preamble to that which I really desired. It was more than a marriage between two people; it was my ticket to establishing a loving family with my new husband, Michael. And we both agreed that we wanted to start this family right away.

I was raised with six brothers and sisters (products of a mixed marriage between a second generation Irish Catholic and an umpteenth generation Daughter of the American Revolution.) Michael was the youngest of five. We were both used to bustling and active households filled with life, laughter, and love and we wanted to replicate that happiness in our own lives. Of course this was long before we actually attempted to raise our three daughters and were forced to buy thongs, finance pedicures, pay for the drama of "Proma", cough up college tuition, and watch our hard-earned money go through the juicing machine – leaving our daughters with only the finest of what we had to offer. But that's a story for another book.

Michael and I would both now freely admit that we were nothing short of naïve as we stood in the church on that glorious day. Perhaps we were simply sanguine, giddy with excitement, or besotted by love, but clearly my new husband and I had no way of knowing the full extent of what parenting would entail. Others around us made it look easy, and our plan was simple. We'd have a couple of beautiful babies. Everyone would "Oooooh" and "Aaaaaah" over them. They, in turn, would grow up to be extremely gifted, exceedingly brilliant, and financially successful enough to take care of us in our old age. Astounding plan, wasn't it?

Who was thinking about challenges back then? Who could foresee that things may not go as planned, especially when external complications came into play? Once we jumped on that child-bearing train we never guessed that we had just entrusted that precious ticket to the ultimate roller coaster attendant.

Family Planning

While Michael and I had the *accepting* children part down pat, it turns out that the *having* children part did not come as smoothly as anticipated. Being the optimist I was, I had no reason to believe that I would encounter the pregnancy problems which eventually came to haunt me. My older sister had endured two successful pregnancies, and my mother had given birth to seven healthy children.

The only glitch in my mother's pregnancies had to do with the reason that the first six of her seven children were born in the French Hospital in New York City instead of the local hospital in northern New Jersey where we were raised. It was a story fit for quirky family annals and I am sure, if tidbits were known, would have set quite a few tongues wagging at my grandparents' respective country clubs.

In 1951, when my mother was first pregnant and living in Tennessee, her obstetrician a routine test for syphilis. Of course the same test had been negative a year earlier when my parents married, but suddenly it was positive.

How could this be? How could this beautiful (and Catholic) debutante have contracted a condition as taboo as this? Now although my father had served in England, not France, in the First World War, several eyes of suspicion immediately came to rest upon him, but his test results were negative. And so my grandparents collectively concluded that an unsanitary southern bathtub in a rented apartment must have been the culprit. My father quickly moved my mother back home to the New York area where an obstetric specialist was found who could deal with this unusual sort of "complication."

I am not quite certain if this particular doctor spent his career delivering babies for wealthy New York socialites with venereal diseases, or if he was on the cutting edge in the field of obstetrics, but somehow he was able to quickly put my parents' fears to rest by assuring them that he had seen many "false-positive" results like hers in pregnant women. His declaration that the results of this test were wrong and that my mother had not contracted the dreaded disease brought a joint sigh of relief from Philadelphia to New York. Nevertheless, my mother continued to have these false-positive findings with each of her successive (and successful) pregnancies. Each time, the results of the same test would return to normal after a baby was born.

The only other red flag that comes to mind is a vivid memory of watching an ambulance pull up our driveway one afternoon shortly after my younger brother was born. As soon as it left with my mother inside, my grandmother marched the five older siblings into our living room and made us stay on our knees for over an hour, praying for our mother's recovery. Our mother had experienced a post-delivery hemorrhage which had sent her back to the local hospital. The earnest prayers of five small children were answered and my mother recovered without incident.

Pregnancies. Babies. Children. My mother had delivered seven of them, and now it was my turn.

Pregnancy Testing

I suppose that back in my mother's day a woman who suspected she was with child went to her doctor for a test which I vaguely recall having something to do with killing a rabbit. (Why any red-blooded obstetrician ever abandoned the earlier test which used mice as their victims instead of cute little bunnies, I'll never know.) But, as we all know, ever since the 1980's a woman can find out at home with something called the *Early Pregnancy Test.*

I am not sure there is another product on the market that has greater power to change a woman's life within ten minutes than an at-home pregnancy test. What's more, rabbit or not, we allow a woman to undergo the emotions intertwined with this test all by herself in her home bathroom without ever speaking with another human being. This is a test of consequence, and women endure the sentiments which come with the outcome of this test in complete obscurity. Have you ever known a woman who casually thought, "Oh, I think I'll take a pregnancy test today?"

As a postmenopausal woman, I freely confess that I have not had the opportunity to use one of these products for more than two decades (and as to whether or not I have found an occasional test stored away in my daughters' bathroom closet, my lips remain sealed) but nonetheless I have a suggestion for those who make them. Instead of having a line system which simply offers the results "Pregnant" or "Not Pregnant" you may want to think about offering a few more options for your users, for the rest of the world does not think simply in binary terms as you appear to do.

We're complicated, and anxious, and emotive. We use your product for many reasons and await your results with diverse sentiments: hopeful anticipation, trepidation, fear of failure, optimism, or reluctance.

You name it, with my crazy, conflicting, and what seemed at the time to be unrelated pregnancy problems, I've been there.

Daughter Number One

If you remember that little wedding question where I

enthusiastically promised to welcome my still yet un-conceived children into this world, I now need to admit that I still thought that this day would come in the not-too-distant future. (Key word here is, "future".) Imagine my shock and dismay when a mere two months after getting married my jeans stopped fitting correctly and total strangers began to ask when I was "due."

"Pregnancy? Impossible!" I pronounced, for I had been bleeding intermittently. And although I railed at the nerve of these meddling people, I finally succumbed to the doubt they implanted by purchasing a new-to-the-market home pregnancy test. Truth be told, I did not purchase just one. In my resolute belief in my non-pregnant state, I secured a two-pack and planned to use them both – the first to prove I was not currently pregnant, and the second for later down the road when that blessed state would arrive according to plan.

I quickly discovered that there is no such thing as a plan when dealing with childbearing because that little pink strip showed that I was indeed pregnant. This shocking fact was confirmed by an obstetrician later in the week and quickly put to the test the following day.

Upon returning home from work, I felt a sharp pain in my abdomen followed by a severe onset of bleeding – so much blood, in fact, that when the doctor first examined me in the emergency room he was convinced that I was experiencing the rupture of a fallopian tube from an ectopic pregnancy. Yet a pre-surgical ultrasound revealed that an intact 12-week-old fetus was contentedly residing in my uterus instead. Yes, I had been pregnant for three months and didn't know it. The best, and most likely, conclusion my doctor could then draw was that the bleeding was due to a miscarriage of a second baby, a twin.

And so with a strange mixture of shock, joy, and grief, my husband and I looked forward to welcoming our new baby shortly before our first wedding anniversary in November.

Until that plan went awry once again.

Would it surprise you to discover that I'm not really much of planner after all? I'd say that procrastinator is the term which better describes me. A mere five weeks before my first child was due to land on this earth, I had not prepared a nursery or purchased one piece of furniture or clothing for this baby. But children, as it turns out, do not care about such necessities when they decide the time has come for them to leave their mother's womb. At a routine 35-week visit on a Friday afternoon my ankles were swollen, my blood pressure was significantly elevated, and there was a trace of protein in my urine. The doctor sent me home with instructions to spend the weekend lying on my left side and return to his office for further monitoring on Monday morning.

While I will admit to being a procrastinator, I have never been a rule breaker, but I took a walk on the wild side that weekend when I got out of bed to attend a baby shower for a friend the following day. (Sitting up or lying down – what's really the difference? I wasn't out playing tennis somewhere!) My water began to break on Saturday evening and our little healthy, but topsy-turvy breach-positioned daughter was born via Caesarian section the following day.

When the moment arrived for me to sit upright and hold my firstborn in my arms for our initial moment of bonding, something went terribly wrong. The room started spinning and I adroitly passed this new bundle of joy off to my husband. I then found myself cradling one of those little hospital throw-up basins instead. Not quite the auspicious start to motherhood I would have hoped for, but a beginning nonetheless. And I quickly discovered that the phrase about payback is all they say it is as this tiny little baby made up for our ignoble first meeting by emptying the contents of her stomach on each and every inch of me for the first three months of her life.

Even though she arrived a full five weeks early, our newborn daughter weighed over seven pounds and was blessedly healthy. Michael and I joyfully named her Kaitlyn and watched the inaugural scene that she and her sisters were destined to re-enact in countless tanning booths during their teenage years, as she lay in the hospital nursery under ultraviolet lights in only diaper and protective goggles to offset her infant jaundice – the sole complication of her early arrival.

After five days in the hospital she and I were free to come home, and we quickly found out how much this new addition to our family liked a party, for she attended her own baby shower the following weekend and was the guest of honor at our first anniversary dinner just two months later.

And how perfect our little bundle was; although looking back at those first pictures, perhaps she was one of those babies that only her parents could love. She had dark brown hair which quickly fell out, leaving her with a ring of hair resembling a monk's tonsure. Her little ear was a bit cauliflowered and crumpled from being scrunched up in the breach position for all that time. And I suppose her neck muscles lacked more than a little strength, because she couldn't hold her head quite straight. The fact that she spent the first six months of her life with her head listing to one side is well documented in the many photos and videos taken by her adoring parents, for she was bone-of-our-bone and flesh-of-our-flesh, and how we loved every quirky bit of her!

I loved being a mother – so much so, that before long I found myself wishing for the opportunity to use that second at-home pregnancy test and discover myself *enceinte* once again.

Daughter Number Two

I didn't get a chance to use that second test for many months running. Although my menstrual period would very frequently be days late, it would eventually appear and my fledgling hopes of another pregnancy would be dashed until the following month. After about eight months, I returned to the obstetrician to work on fertility issues. At the conclusion of a series of painful prodding, humiliating testing, daily temperature taking, and less-than-spontaneous attempts at conceiving, I was placed on a fertility drug and four months later the second, perhaps-slightly-expired, pregnancy test was at last used with successful results. How beautiful it would be to have two children – one for each hand I dreamily thought. And, although our children would be spaced approximately three years apart, we had only lost about eighteen months in our quest to build our family.

This time all remained uneventful until I arrived at a doctor's visit on yet another Friday afternoon four weeks before my due date, when once again my blood pressure was elevated and protein was found in my urine. This time I was told to report to the hospital the next morning for a fetal stress test. When I arrived, it was evident that I was in the early stages of toxemia (pre-eclampsia) and our second daughter was quickly delivered by Cesarean section shortly after noon.

Megan, like most toxemic babies, was tiny for her gestational age but healthy despite her 4 pound, 8 ounce weight. I don't remember if they calculated an Apgar score on her, but from the wail that came out of her upon her first breath in her new world, there was no doubt that her lungs were fully formed. Remembering the first nauseating encounter with Kaitlyn, I don't think I even attempted to raise my body to a sitting position to hold her until I knew I had regained my sea legs once again.

Like her sister before her, Megan was ready to leave the hospital with me five days later, but this time there were restrictions placed upon our comings and goings. For the next four weeks, Megan and her newly-discovered vocal chords were only allowed to leave the house to go to the pediatrician's office. While she may not have been the happiest baby ever put on the planet, Megan was still our longed-for child and we lovingly put up with her distrust of sleep and colicky crying. And despite my best effort to avoid insulting my new daughter by not throwing up on her at our first face-to-face meeting, it turns out that she did not bother to return the compliment and instead surpassed her older sister in her proclivity for projectile vomiting.

Now I ask you, with all of this happy domesticity who wouldn't want to add some more by having another child? And when it took months of trying and the help of fertility drugs to sustain a pregnancy the last time, why not begin the process sooner rather than later?

And that is precisely why our third daughter, Leah, was born just 17 months after her sister Megan.

Daughter Number Three

I suppose by this time I should have given up all thoughts of the oxymoron, "family planning" but some people appear destined to repeat the same mistakes over and over again. Being greeted with yet-another shock at the rapidity at which my third pregnancy overtook me, I quickly marched myself to the obstetrician with a "What now?" look upon my face. I cannot say that I was really concerned for my health, although the pre-eclampsia episode would have scared a saner individual. I think I was just at a loss as to why this "accepting children lovingly from God" thing was so unpredictable. Why could I conceive when I wasn't quite trying and not conceive when I was? Why did these babies not want to stay and grow to full-term? Was I doing something wrong? Were Michael and I somehow incompatible in the childbearing department?

At this appointment my obstetrician told me that there had been some new discoveries about pregnancies like mine. I now remember him referring to my body fighting against itself and viewing what I mistakenly assumed was the fetus as a foreign invader. This, he explained, was why I had trouble sustaining my pregnancies and also accounted for the pre-eclampsia and early labor I had experienced. He also told me that the medical community had reported some success placing patients with my condition on low-dose aspirin and monitoring them more closely. I left the office that day, still more than a bit bewildered. "So much for the bone-of-my-bone and flesh-of-my-flesh," I thought. "Could it be true that my body was turning on my own children? What kind of unnatural mother was I?"

Natural or unnatural, I didn't have time to dwell much on these new thoughts, as I had two small children by the hand (I don't know where I thought I was going to put the third) and Megan was barely nine-months old. I took that aspirin dutifully each morning and prayed for the best. I was even encouraged when I experienced morning sickness for the first time. "Perhaps this pregnancy will be the normal one," I hoped. And by this time I had so much dislike for unplanned events that I begged my doctor to schedule a C-section a few days before my due date in January because I was tired of subjecting myself to the fickleness of fate.

They say a tiger can't change his stripes, so I suppose it would be silly to think that fate could shed her fickleness. In reality, I am not quite sure if any of the laws of nature applied to me when I was with child, for I went into labor just four days after Christmas and our third daughter, Leah, was born via C-section after hours of "unproductive" labor. Despite the nomenclature, this third pregnancy seemed the most productive to me. My pregnancy itself lasted almost a full week longer than the other two. Leah was a healthy baby, weighing in at six pounds, four ounces, and I had remained healthy right up to the pre-mature end – a victory of sorts for me. Still, I knew that this pregnancy would be my last, for my doctor, husband, and I all agreed the time had come to stop tempting the fertility gods.

Leah, too, declared victory and made it part of her life plan to dispel that "unproductive" label. While Leah was – by nature – a happy baby, she was clearly different from the other two. Struggling to keep up with her older sisters, she walked and talked much earlier than they had. She developed a keen knowledge of the world around her and a fierce sense of competition. As she was dragged to choir concerts, soccer practice, and gymnastics lessons along with the older two, this tenacious toddler quickly discovered that she did not like watching life from the sidelines. Leah yearned to be an active participant. That product of my unproductive labor studied how the older children spoke, looked, and acted and then carefully created her own "to do" list.

And so, after the birth of our third child, I put the mysterious childbearing chapter of my life behind me, thankful for the gift of three beautiful and healthy daughters – despite all of my problems in getting them here.

It wasn't until years later, when I read a chapter in a book written by my daughters' rheumatologist, that the term "antiphospholipid antibody syndrome" put those puzzle pieces together for me; for this syndrome provokes pregnancy-related complications such as miscarriage, stillbirth, preterm delivery, and pre-eclampsia. That very same chapter also shed light on the results of my mother's pregnancy blood tests. In what may seem to be a quirky coincidence, it turns out that a "false positive" result on a syphilis test is an indication that one type of these antibodies is present in your system. In my mother's case they caused no harm and disappeared once she was no longer pregnant, but the concept itself was intriguing to me while trying to understand my own pregnancy challenges.

2. The Early Years

Don't cry because it's over.
Smile because it happened.

– Dr. Seuss

Despite what all those parenting books tell you, the first years of motherhood are quite simple. Forget the hype about the loss of sleep, horrors of temper tantrums, and the endless chasing of toddlers; that stuff is easy. You may encounter some cuts and bruises along the way, but no one ever said that mothering was for the faint of heart.

In a move of sheer coincidence, my husband recently pulled out some old videos from when our daughters were young, and we have spent time viewing them together as a family. Witnessing the cheerful spontaneity and joy that our children possessed in those days makes my heart yearn to live them all over again. Let me pause to relate one little life-story documented on these videos:

The scene is Easter morning and the father is filming the annual Easter egg hunt in the spinning household. Based on many an outcry that the mother of the family has adjudicated in the past, she gets all of the wee folk to agree that once the hunt is over she will ensure that the outcome is fair and equitable to all. Once the starting gate is opened, all three of those daughters run with wild abandon, attempting to find those eggs. The youngest child, prancing around in a chiffon bathrobe, seems more determined than the rest but yet complains that she isn't finding as many as her older sisters. Believing that the dear child is correct, the bunny who actually hid the eggs while her husband slept blissfully upstairs, directs the child with a hint or two.

Once the hunt is declared officially over and the interested parties sit on the living room floor, all eggs are then counted by their respective finders. The count comes in as follows: Kaitlyn, the oldest, has collected eight eggs. Megan, the middle, has nabbed nine. Leah, the youngest, has somehow managed to accumulate ten of those jelly-filled wonders. The mother of the house (who may just feel as if she's been played for a fool by her three-year-old offspring) feels strongly that fairness between her daughters is important. Listen carefully as each daughter attempts to attain this equity in her own way:

Kaitlyn quickly begins to gather all the eggs into one pile and redistribute them evenly. Great try on her part, but the mother stops her, for she has decided to turn this particular moment in to a math-generosity lesson. Kaitlyn then happily sits back, trusting in her parents' promise to make all things right.

Megan then has a wonderfully magnanimous idea. She decides that the best way to handle the inequity is for the excess eggs to be given to her parents so that each of the sisters will possess eight eggs. Lovely in its generous inception, but not quite fulfilling the math equation her mother is looking for.

The camera pans to Leah who quips, "Oh, I know!" She then proceeds to handle one of her precious eggs and immediately does an about-face, declaring, "Never mind!" Prodded on by her mother, she puts aside what she views as one of her hard-earned eggs and yet – no matter how many times she counts those eggs remaining in front of her – still continues to count ten in her collection. Clearly, there is no way of getting around this poor child's possession of ten eggs!

How I wish I were astute enough at that time to realize how those five minutes of bunny droppings reflected the ultimate personalities of all of those in our little family unit. Kaitlyn, an eternal optimist, knows instinctively that it will all turn out right in the end and is willing to wait it out without protest or tears. Megan, generous to a fault, is willing to give away what she and her sister possess. Leah, as the youngest, has already learned that survival in this world needs to come with a touch of tenacity and fuzzy math. That fuzzy math will come to her aid many times in the future as she tries to explain away her multiple purchases at the mall as a teenager.

Were any of them wrong, or better, than the other? Of course not. Leah, before long, saw the wisdom in giving her older sister that which she was lacking. Megan was duly praised for her generous offer. And Kaitlyn's heart was reaffirmed by the fact that trust and optimism win out in the end.

The truth is that once my childbearing years were behind me, I had thrown myself whole-heartedly into raising these children. If, by chance, I had not been so natural in producing them, I certainly made up for it in mothering them. I had stopped working just before our second daughter, Megan, was born and so had the time and unlimited energy to devote to them. Thinking that we had at last jumped off that roller coaster, we then chugged through life's ups-and-downs with ease: baby teeth, ear infections, stomach bugs, chicken pox, speech therapy, braces, broken bones, strep infections, and even a case of hand, foot, and mouth disease.

But through it all, it was Megan who claimed the biggest piece of the motherhood worrying pie. Megan was the child who spent the first five years of her life with a perpetual cold. Megan was the one who needed speech therapy at the age of three. Megan was the daughter who displayed a touch of ADHD. She was the student the teachers suggested repeat kindergarten a second year. Megan was the one who, by second grade, had been diagnosed with a learning disability. It was Megan who experienced terrible growing pains at night. Megan, who walked on tiptoe and needed physical therapy to allow the muscles in her legs to keep up with her growing bones. Megan was the daughter who needed glasses and was susceptible to cavities although her sisters had never heard a dentist's drill or sat in an ophthalmologist's chair.

It wasn't that Megan was all that different from my other daughters; it's just that I could not help but think, "Why do these things keep happening to Megan?" Was it a presentiment? Mother's intuition? A sense of foreboding? I honestly cannot say.

The fact is that all three of my daughters lived active and happy lives – with endless rounds of gymnastics sessions, soccer games, basketball practices, and Irish dancing lessons. It's not that we were without the occasional visit to the doctor, but I wasn't one to dwell on any physical ailments.

To this day, my children still chuckle at the fact that I wouldn't bring them to the doctor unless they were dying. They make fun of me for the time I made Kaitlyn attempt to complete her homework in the radiologist's waiting room three full days after she had injured her right wrist in a bicycle accident. The homework became irrelevant the minute the technician came out to announce that her wrist was indeed broken. They laugh just remembering the pediatrician's reaction when I finally brought Megan to the office one long week after she had been hobbling around on one foot. When I mentioned the fact that the foot didn't seem swollen to me, the indignant doctor replied "What do you mean? It's swollen like crazy!"

I am going to state for the record that it was not my fault

when Megan alone made the decision to continue to dance a four-hand reel in the Northeastern regional Irish dancing competition despite the fact that she had broken her foot five minutes before while practicing backstage. Even I recognized the fact that it was "swollen like crazy" and sent her off to the closest Philadelphia hospital with my husband while I stayed to watch Leah dance in the next competition. And I did not hesitate to call 911 (that is, after I called my mother) the day that Kaitlyn fell down a full flight of stairs in our home and ended up sprawled at the bottom with a bone clearly sticking out of her left arm. And I willingly accompanied her in yet another ambulance just three weeks after that first cast came off when she tripped on a boardwalk and broke her other arm.

Perhaps my ultimate pride in motherhood lies in the fact that I insisted on dragging Leah to the emergency room against her will with what I knew were the unmistakable signs of appendicitis. Leah was, and always will be, the child who insists she isn't sick; but I had experienced appendicitis which wasn't caught right away at exactly her age and, consequently, spent five weeks in the hospital getting rid of the peritoneal infection. I didn't have to watch that child's attempt to stagger towards the bathroom for long before I recognized the pain she was in and was not going to let that little episode repeat itself with one of my daughters. If you do not yet believe that we were a normal, all-American family, I offer you just a few of the other childhood crises my family endured without missing a beat:

> **The time** my mother took three-year-old Kaitlyn to the grocery store, and she then proceeded to sit in the carriage and sing, "*My Daddy drinks beer and I like to pick my nose!*"

> **The day** the very same child came home from first grade with a note informing me that she had told her religion

teacher that her mother, *"Really liked to drink the wine at church."*

The oh-so-proud day Megan fell off the end of the second row of risers at her kindergarten graduation, causing the teachers to sandwich her in the middle when she graduated again the following year.

The afternoon five-year-old Leah yelled repeatedly at the attendant on the "Froggy" ride demanding that he, *"Stop this thing, I'm gonna throw up!"* She then reprimanded her own mother for being powerless to speak because she was laughing too hard, leaving the terrified child to take matters into her own hands.

The countless times Megan's trigger finger, which remained stuck in the open position when she closed her hand, would be utilized to point at things. The only problem with this was that this particular finger happened to be her middle finger. *"Oh, look, there's a bird!"*

The time we took Kaitlyn to the neurologist after her science teacher expressed concern that she was experiencing seizures during class, only to come out with a firm diagnosis of daydreaming.

The day Leah attempted to jump out of Michael's moving car because she hated first grade.

And then there was the time Megan, when asked by the child study team to list the three things she wished for most, answered *"Happiness and World Peace."* If you had those two, why would you ever need a third?

Have I convinced you yet that I was a rational and level-headed mother? Well I was. I knew I was going to need every ounce of sanity as we headed into those girl's teenage years. And those years were fast approaching; for in the blink of an eye Kaitlyn turned 13 and went off to high school. The others were just a few short years behind her.

Intertwined with the tumultuous teenage whirlwind came a whole other host of health nightmares as my daughters traded those childhood bruises, breaks, and braces for far more nightmarish terms like antibodies, anemia, and arthritis.

3. Lupus

It all began with a shoe on the wall.
A shoe on the wall shouldn't be there at all.

– Dr. Seuss

The Pigtail Precursor

Looking back now with the prescience that hindsight brings, I believe I can date the first signs of Megan's illness to her preschool years. As you may have already guessed, Megan was one of those children who experienced life just a little bit differently. Part of this difference was the fact that she had always been acutely attuned to external stimuli.

I am not sure that Megan ever really slept until she entered her teenage years. As an infant, when she would finally succumb to that slumbering state my husband and I so longed for, we learned that we could never enter the room to check on her, for no matter how stealthily we tiptoed up to her crib, the slightest movement would cause her to awaken and spring up from sleep. One day, when she was nine years old, I found clock times penciled on the wall by her bedside. When asked, she told me that she had begun to document all of the different times she was awake throughout the night.

If you chanced to peek into her room and actually find her asleep in her bed, she would invariably be lying on her back in a corpse-like stance – proof that she had never attempted to settle in to a cozy night's sleep, but stayed awake battling the feeling until sleep finally took her unawares.

One of my favorite stories as a child was the fairy tale, *The Princess and the Pea*. I always imagined Megan as that princess who could feel the presence of the tiniest pea even though the mattresses were stacked 50 deep. Megan never liked any excess of physical sensations. I suppose if her mother were more than a tad bit thinner, Megan would have been the perfect candidate to be raised in a nudist colony, for she wore dresses only (one particular favorite over and over again) would not bear the thought of tights against her skin, and made me turn her socks inside-out because she couldn't stand the stitching along the toe line.

If Megan had her dislikes, she had her loves too. Have I told you how much she loved the color yellow? Megan was enthralled with yellow and wanted to surround herself in it. I suppose that's how she acquired that sunny disposition which became so apparent throughout her teenage years. One thing I do know for sure is that the color yellow is the reason she shares her mother's unnatural love of all-things-cheese to this day.

Megan could not stand the sensation of having her hair brushed either, but yet she insisted on wearing her blond hair in pigtails. Of course the configuration of these pigtails involved parting her hair with a single line from her forehead to the nape of her neck. When she was three years old I noticed some questionable areas developing on the crown of her head (See, I told you she was a princess!) right along the part line. Two distinct disk-shaped lesions began to appear and, worse yet, her hair began to fall out from these lesions and didn't seem to want to grow back. Being the attentive mother we have already discovered I was in those days, I marched my splotchy-headed-yellow-clad daughter to the dermatologist who diagnosed her with eczema and gave me cream and shampoo to use on her. Neither one helped to clear up the lesions and, much to my embarrassment, Megan continued to insist on putting her ugly bald spots on display for all to see.

You may not know this little fact regarding suburban pre-school life, but in those days competition to have the perfectly-clad child was fierce between mothers. Other children would show up for school flawlessly clothed, socked, and coiffed with bows in their hair. But, try as I might, Megan would appear at school in her favorite yellow dress, socks inside-out, with two big spots gleaming from her head – for there simply wasn't a bow big enough to cover them.

Eight years later, as I frantically began to read about the manifestations of this disease called lupus, I realized that these lesions may have been an outward precursor to the systemic disease itself. As I watched with tears as her hair fell out in droves, I knew then that this was not just a childhood illness. It was an illness that would be with her for life.

But I am getting ahead of myself here.

"Like" Lupus

We need to return to the very Christmas Eve when Megan was eleven years old and woke up with the unmistakable signs of a strep throat infection. Perhaps she woke up with them the day before and in my Christmas frenzy I put the doctor's visit off in hopes that it would go away, but any red-blooded mother would have done the same and then panicked, knowing that no help would be in sight on

Christmas Day itself. Sure enough, the swab tested at the pediatrician's office turned positive and they placed Megan on a ten day regimen of antibiotics which lasted through the beginning of the New Year. Although she appeared to improve at first, a few days after finishing her last dose of the antibiotic she became sick again with the same symptoms, leading us back to the pediatrician's office for round two and yet-another positive test for the streptococcal bacteria.

I have since heard it said that the very definition of insanity is the repeating of an action and assuming it will bring a different outcome. If so, I can no longer attest to my slight hold on sanity because I became an unwitting bystander in a vicious cycle of no less than six "deja vu" antibiotic treatments. The only difference was that Megan became sicker with each relapse. By February she began complaining of leg and joint pain and started hobbling around the house. In March, we could no longer rouse her from her now-established squatter's rights on her parents' bed, spending every daylight hour watching the *Animal Planet* channel on television; her innate love of animals being the only interest still left in her life.

And school? The cycle here repeated itself with disastrous results. Megan would be well enough to attend school for only a day or two before a relapse would send her back home to life on Animal Planet. It is not as though I did not voice my growing concern during our repeated visits to the various doctors in our pediatric practice, but we rarely saw the same physician twice. One ran some blood work and nothing seemed out of whack. Another was sure it was Osgood-Schlatter Disease and referred us to our good friends at the orthopedic group where, because of the myriad of previous broken bones, we were already known on a first name basis. At last someone had the presence of mind to run a blood test which I had never heard the likes of before. He called it a "sed" rate, which I later learned was officially called an Erythrocyte Sedimentation Rate (ESR). A final doctor, upon seeing that the sed rate was significantly elevated (a sign that inflammation may be occurring somewhere in her body) ordered a test for Antinuclear Antibodies (ANA) which subsequently came back positive.

Antinuclear Antibodies? I now look back in wonder at my naiveté regarding this nomenclature. Was there really a time when I didn't know what an antinuclear antibody portended? The pediatrician tried to explain what he knew and referred us to a pediatric rheumatologist at a larger hospital a half-hour away. I also quickly learned that the term "pediatric rheumatologist" was practically an oxymoron, since most rheumatologic issues, like arthritis, affect older adults. In fact, I still remember the pediatrician telling me that a convention of pediatric rheumatologists could be held in an intimate French restaurant – his way of letting me know that the incidence of pediatric issues was so rare that there were not many physicians who treated the pediatric population. These issues may be rare, but serious, I learned.

Michael and I waited for that first visit to the rheumatologist with bated breath, for although her bouts with strep throat had finally come to an end, Megan was no longer well enough to even attempt a day at school and was receiving at-home services from the school district. Eventually the big day arrived; the day when I first heard the word "lupus" used in conjunction with my child. The rheumatologist sent Megan for a series of more diagnostic testing – ultrasound and echocardiogram, x-rays and blood work. In the meantime, she prescribed an anti-malarial drug called plaquenil which she explained would begin to help with Megan's fatigue and joint pain.

Can you imagine the euphoria of two worried parents upon

the reception of a lone pill that they hoped would cure their daughter of a plague which had visited her for over four months? I still shudder at the disenchantment I experienced when, after picking up the precious medicine, I read the insert which stated, "If you don't see results after six months on this medicine consult your physician."

Six months? Did they really mean six months? What kind of a long haul were we in for?

It was the discovery that Megan was producing way too many new red blood cells – a condition called Hemolytic Anemia – which, along with her joint pain and other irregular findings in her bloodwork, caused this rheumatologist to definitively diagnose Megan with lupus and prescribe the steroid, prednisone. I am still, to this day, ashamed to admit that I had no idea of what an autoimmune disease was at that time.

When life sends you disappointment, an optimistic person believes there are always second chances and we believed ours would come in the form of a second opinion. In this vein, our pediatrician secured us an appointment with the Chief of Pediatric Rheumatology at one of the big hospitals in New York City who was alleged to be the premier pediatric rheumatologist on the East Coast. By the time this doctor first saw Megan she had responded to the prednisone treatment ordered by the first rheumatologist and was in relatively good shape.

After his extensive blood tests and physical exam, he rescinded the previous doctor's diagnosis of lupus. Yes, it looked like lupus, smelled like lupus, and even walked and talked like lupus, but in the absence of serious systemic manifestations, like kidney issues, he would not definitively diagnose her with the disease. Rheumatologic conditions and autoimmune diseases, he explained, were tough to label since so many symptoms overlap and mimic each other. Even those antibodies which were clearly present in Megan's blood are not always specific, and sometimes can act as red herrings. In fact, lupus is sometimes called "The Great Imitator" because its symptoms are often like the symptoms of other rheumatologic and autoimmune diseases. It is not the label that matters after all, he said, but the treatment plan. And so he began to treat her as if she had lupus, but has since – in the ensuing fifteen years – watched her disease activity closely and kept an eye out for other diseases.

And if, by chance, her rheumatologist wasn't watching, have no fear. I was. I read and studied each and every aspect of her disease. I learned how to zero in on blood test results faster than a SWAT team member at target practice. I followed her sed rate CRP (C reactive protein) complements, and her double-stranded-anti-DNA like a crime scene investigator. I kept her exposure to the sun at a bare minimum and avoided all other things thought to trigger lupus flares: garlic and alfalfa sprouts, hair coloring and paint thinners. I learned to watch for symptoms of funny sounding overlapping illnesses like Sjogren's Syndrome and Raynaud's phenomenon.

A helicopter parent? Not exactly. More like a submarine sleuth. I wanted to become informed so I could advocate for my child. And now I will share just some of what that sleuthing taught me.

Lupus is a chronic autoimmune disease that can cause damage to almost any part of the body. As we will see is the case with all autoimmune processes, in lupus something goes wrong with the part of the body that fights off foreign invaders like viruses, bacteria, and germs. Normally our immune system produces antibodies which are called up to protect the body from these invaders. When someone has an "autoimmune disease" it means the body's immune system cannot tell the difference between these foreign invaders and the body's healthy tissue and continues to create antibodies even though there is no longer cause. These antibodies then cause the tissues in the body to be in a state of consistent inflammation and produce symptoms like joint pain, muscle pain, and skin rashes.

Perhaps a polite author would use the euphemism, "too much of a good thing" when describing the autoimmune process, but I can't help but think of it as an immune system "run amok" instead.

Lupus is also a disease of flares (the symptoms worsen and you feel ill) and remissions (the symptoms improve and you feel better.) Lupus is not the same disease for all people and can range from mild to life-threatening. A wide range of symptoms may come and go, popping up at different times during the course of the disease. Damage from lupus can also cause serious and life-threatening conditions in brain, heart, kidney, and liver functions.

Most lupus patients are women who first develop symptoms while in their childbearing years. Less than one percent of the 1.5 million Americans with lupus are diagnosed while under the age of 18. How was it that the symptoms of this serious disease began to manifest themselves in my yellow-clad-pigtail-girl despite these odds?

While, thankfully, Megan has not experienced any serious complications from her illness, the most worrisome part of her story has been the discovery that Megan, too, tests positive for those antiphospholipid antibodies which her grandmother and I most likely encountered during our pregnancies. Approximately 50 percent of people with lupus have these antibodies circulating in their blood, yet as we have seen, people without lupus can have them too. Sometimes they come and go, increase and decrease. Along with pregnancy complications, the presence of these antibodies is associated with a predisposition for blood clots which can form anywhere in the body. Serious stuff.

For the most part, Megan has been able to enjoy what others would view a normal life. Although she experienced two painful bouts with pleurisy, she finished the rest of her junior high years without incident then stormed her way through the drama and turmoil of her high school years – using those vocal chords to dish out barbs to her mother like a pitcher in major league baseball. She also threw herself with gusto into sorority life upon entering college and graduated with a B.S. in Psychology after four years. Upon graduation, Megan got a job as a vision therapist and rarely missed a day of work for health reasons.

Although Megan suffers from joint pain and fatigue every day of her life, her pain is mitigated somewhat by prescription Non Steroidal Anti Inflammatory Drugs (NSAIDs) and a new biologic medication she takes. Every once in a while her symptoms or blood test results demand that she go on a low dose of steroids, but because long term use of steroids can cause bone erosion and additional medical problems, she always makes it a priority to taper off as soon as possible.

She's lucky. We feel blessed. The disease has never caused damage to any of her major organs or systems. Yet she's young and admittedly has a lifetime of unknown challenges ahead.

4. Spondyloarthropathies

From there to here,
from here to there,
funny things are everywhere.

– Dr. Seuss

You recall that I have three daughters in total. Thus far I have focused on my middle daughter, Megan, and her battle with her lupus-like illness. One sick daughter would have been bad enough, but that doesn't mean that the other two would escape unscathed, for they, too, have dealt with their own health issues.

Not long after Megan was diagnosed-undiagnosed-but-treated as if she had lupus, Leah began complaining about pain in her heels when she danced. A word of explanation here: My one regret from my childhood was that I never got the chance to learn Irish step dancing like others in my grammar school class. Those were the days when the "Lace Curtain Irish" were moving away from the customs and traditions of the old sod. I didn't care which kind of curtains we had hanging in our living room, I had come down with a debilitating case of costume envy. I yearned to wear those fancy dresses and have my curly hair bob up and down with each step. Why was I forced to wear refined ballet slippers when my classmates were sporting their lace-up ghillies? And so, thirty years later, I watched as my daughters lived out my childhood fantasy – complete with elaborate attire, special wigs (yes, wigs!) and fancy shoes.

Not so bad, really. They loved it. And I gleefully paid for, and drove them to, dance class two or three times a week and enrolled them in dance competitions once a month. The Irish call each competition a feis, but it was really an opportunity to dress them up and collect various trophies which have been long-relegated to basement boxes.

But their ankles, knees, and heels took a real beating. Kaitlyn was now in high school and so was no longer interested in dance and Megan's dancing days ended with the onset of her joint pain. Leah was my last connection to my unrequited childhood passion and loved those jigs and reels almost as much as I did. Unsurprisingly, she also reveled in the competition and her collection of trophies. When she started complaining about her heels hurting, I assumed it was some sort of overuse injury and took her to the ever-friendly orthopedist who quickly diagnosed her heel pain as Sever's disease – inflammation of the heel's growth plate usually caused by overuse and stress on the heel bone. Weird sounding? Yes. But I was starting to learn a lot about these eponymous diseases and conditions. And, despite its name, this wasn't a disease. It was a condition easily cured by rest and physical therapy.

Phew.

Unfortunately Leah's pain did not subside with rest and physical therapy and she started to complain about other joints hurting as well. There ended Leah's dancing career and my vicarious fascination with all things Irish.

At around the same time, Kaitlyn began complaining about pain in her hips when playing lacrosse. (Disclaimer: sweating on a lacrosse team wearing ugly blue and gold uniforms with my hair in braids was not one of my childhood fantasies.) Before long, the discomfort began to creep into other areas as well and she experienced pain and swelling in her joints. Normally possessed of a joyful and optimist spirit, I knew that when Kaitlyn complained I needed to listen.

Believe me when I tell you that some of this remains a blur to me and I am not exactly sure whether it was Leah or Kaitlyn who developed this type of pain first, but the end result was that we ended up with a family discount in the rheumatologist's office because all three of our offspring became patients within a year of each other.

Unlike their sister, none of the extensive blood tests run showed any abnormalities, but the pain, swelling and tenderness were obvious. They were each diagnosed with something called a spondyloarthropapathy and placed on NSAIDs.

Relief. Yet now I had to learn all about this odd sounding condition.

I am immeasurably thankful that their rheumatologist, Dr. Thomas Lehman, authored a book on childhood joint pain and rheumatic diseases. His book, *It's Not Just Growing Pains* has been my "go to" book ever since it was published in 2004. We were already regular patients by that time, but the chapters on lupus, spondyloarthropathies, Raynaud's phenomenon, Sjogren's Syndrome, and laboratory and diagnostic testing have been invaluable tools to me as different symptoms and issues have since popped into my family members' lives.

So, with the help of Dr. Lehman's book, I will attempt to explain this strange sounding condition. Spondyloarthropathy is a pattern of arthritis that can crop up for any number of underlying reasons. Pain around the joint is the hallmark symptom. Much of the pain involved comes from tendonitis around the wrists, knees, ankles, or heels.

While some children with this pattern of arthritis have specific underlying issues which explain their pain and discomfort, many children (like mine) have a nonspecific onset. Some will go on to develop psoriasis or inflammatory bowel disease later in life which will explain the earlier arrival of arthritis, but many will remain unchanged for the rest of their lives.

Interestingly enough, when one child has this condition it is common for other family members to be affected as well – another detail that would further obfuscate Megan's lupus/non-lupus diagnosis.

Standard treatment is to be placed on NSAIDs and followed closely by a rheumatologist to make sure that no other issues appear around the bend.

Only God knows how hard I prayed that no more troubles were looming around that bend.

5. Life Despite It All

Today you are You, that is truer than true.
There is no one alive who is Youer than You.

– Dr. Seuss

I understand that I sound somewhat light-hearted when talking about my children's illnesses. Let me assure you that, although I may sound flippant at times, watching my daughters struggle with their respective illnesses was, and continues to be, painful for me. It's tough. It's tragic. It is nothing short of heart wrenching. And although I relate only my own feelings in this book, I know that it has been equally distressing for my husband, Michael, as well.

It would be impossible to tell you how many sleepless nights I have spent worrying about my daughters' health. Nor can I describe the feelings that go through my head when watching them trade painkillers and compare swollen joints, fatigue, and muscle pain. All three. Really? For the rest of their lives?

This is, by no means, fair. Why them? Is it my fault? Is this related to my pregnancy issues? Remember they said I was rejecting those children. . . Why not me? My husband? Or their cousins or friends? Why does every other child seem healthy and carefree?

Will something worse happen? Will they ever be able to lead full and carefree lives? How will I let them go off to college? Get a job? Move away?

There really are no words to relate the angst which I tend to go through. Who can tell me there is anything worse than watching a child grow sicker by the day and have no answers for it? Yes, I was spared the anxiety of the unknown with both Kaitlyn and Leah, for I knew the right direction to go with them, but that was only thanks to the journey undertaken with Megan.

It may be true that hindsight is always 20/20, but as I look back on those horrible first dawnings of illness (and other rude awakenings which were yet to come) I can't help but second guess my actions. Why wasn't I more proactive? More vocal or demanding? Why did I sit back time and time again, only to hear the nurse declare that Megan's strep test was positive? How on earth did I lie next to her, day after day, watching *Animal Planet* on television and not bark at the doctors? Howl at her condition? Roar for more testing?

The best answer I can give is that answers came slowly. Each day brought new challenges, new symptoms, new phone calls, and a new round of waiting for doctor's appointments or test results – leaving me in a constant state of anticipation for the next answer. Unfortunately, the answers received usually were fuzzy, uncertain, and demanded a further round of testing. And incredible as it sounds, I somehow learned to live with uncertainty.

Besides, there were bigger fish to fry in our household. My daughters were entering their teenage years.

Tumultuous Teens

I believe I could fill an entire book on the very topic of my daughters' teenage years, and yet somehow I look at my very same offspring today and think, "What wonderful daughters I have!"

Are females mercifully wired to forget the torment and turmoil that became a part of everyday life while these creatures lived under our roofs? Or, because I endured shortened pregnancies and escaped the pain of childbirth (although the searing sensation of having your insides opened via Caesarian section was no easy feat either) did fate throw extra challenges my way after the fact? I have often thought that I gave birth to each child no less than three times – once to the infant, another to that stranger who appeared about 13 years later, and a final time to that exquisite butterfly who emerged from within her turbulent teenaged cocoon.

During those blissful days when my daughters were young I distinctly remember running into a whole host of older woman in the produce aisle of the grocery story looking wistfully at the small children dangling off the sides of my cart. They would invariably tell me to cherish these years because they would prove to be the best of my life. I mistakenly thought that they were talking about the days when my children would be grown, out of the house, and living full lives of their own. I could not help but long for the day when I wouldn't have to hire a babysitter simply to have dinner with my husband. I couldn't squelch the envy that arose when I spied other women sitting on the beach reading, or shopping alone, or simply crossing the street by themselves.

Then came the day when I realized the truth. Those women who stopped me weren't nostalgic over the loss of children who had grown up and moved away. They were in the throes of raising teenage daughters! I remember that day well, for it was the day that my oldest declared that she no longer wanted me to chaperone the seventh grade class trip to the Museum of Natural History. Did I really try to run her over with the car? I doubt it; although she tells a convincing story. What was that girl thinking? I had devoted the last thirteen years of my life to nurturing and caring for her, and now she didn't want me anywhere near her? Thank the good Lord I had two replacements for her at home.

It turns out that those replacements grow up also. Not only does your precious Snow White get her driver's license, but before you know it her little dwarfs have transformed overnight into Weepy, Creepy, Spendy, Trendy, Needy, Greedy and, let's be nice and call her "Witchy." And don't you think they can't run through each of these personas in the course of a single day, leaving you to wonder if you need to call the pediatrician to report that your daughter is suffering from a multiple personality disorder. It is time to face the cold hard facts that the days of fairy tales and merry-go-rounds, have turned into the dark days of tall tales and real-life bumper cars.

Although most of the years which encompassed my daughters' teenage drama remain a whirlwind of tampons, tofu and twizzlers, if you are still of the mindset of providing a soundtrack for my life at that time, I have a few suggestions for you. I would encourage you to play Eric Clapton's cover of *Lies, Lies, Lies,* along with Santana's *You've Got to Change Your Evil Ways.* Don't forget to add Tommy Roe's *Dizzy* and Blood, Sweat & Tears *Spinning Wheel.* As a matter of fact, you can include anything by Blood, Sweat & Tears because – if you were to only add the word "Cash" to the name of the band – that's exactly what I gave those girls.

Raising teenagers is never an easy task, but it becomes especially problematical when your progeny happens to look like mine: Kaitlyn, with her long dark hair and bright blue eyes, the one with "the map of Ireland on her face," has a vibrant smile and a magnetic happiness. Megan's soft brown hair and expressive blue eyes serve as an alluring window to her reflective and reserved soul. And Leah's sea green eyes and exotic beauty elicit a bit of a "wow" response from all who see her. Slim, attractive, and appealing, all three of my daughters were an invitation for drama to be played out in those years between the age of 13 and 20.

Luckily for all, I kept a sort of diary (i.e. long-abandoned blog) which documented my daughters' teenage years so I am able to relate just a few of these blissful memories to you:

> **How about life before** the word "unlimited" was used in conjunction with cell phone plans? Can you imagine the turmoil created when Megan sent 4,032 texts messages in one month at ten cents a text?

> **Can I ever forget** two of my daughters' unauthorized use of my credit cards? Just imagine what fun they must have had meeting in the mall, swapping those cards between themselves, even buying their friends gifts as tokens of their reckless behavior. What I wouldn't pay to get a glimpse of the mall security films for that day!

> **And how about** the introduction of adhesive breast forms (or "sticky boobs" as I refer to them) instead of old fashioned bras? Was it our dog Kasey's fault that she happens to be a retriever and loved to store my daughters' boobs away in the back of her crate, leaving them covered in pet fur when my daughters needed them? I, for one, applaud the dog's efforts. At least their father and I weren't the only ones who wanted those girls to dress modestly from time to time.

Can you imagine the first time I came up empty-handed when searching the linen closet for a clean bath towel, only to discover 27 of those one-hit-wonders adorning the floors of my daughters' bedrooms?

And how about learning how to drive? I'll never forget the first time I set Megan and her newly-earned driver's license free in a rainstorm. Turns out her silly parents had neglected to teach her anything about the existence of a defrost button. Did she not think she would have noticed if the rest of the world drove with their heads hanging out of the driver's seat window every time it rained?

And the food?

Kaitlyn was the first of my offspring to become a vegetarian. During her high school years, Kaitlyn had the misfortune of working after school in a chiropractor's office where some fool taught her the concept of healthy eating. Sure, I may have gained a few free stabs at cracking her arthritic back, but I lost the ability to ever feed that child macaroni and cheese again. Megan's love of everything-animal was the next to rear its head and so she quickly followed in her sister's vegetarian footsteps, although she never could shake her desire for all-things-dispensed-from-vending-machines. Leah, too, left the meat-eating realm and started demanding healthy and meat-free dinners.

How can I possibly begin to tell you about the money spent attempting to maintain my daughters in the manner that their best friends had come to expect? Aside from the occasional twenty dollar bill regularly lifted from their mother's wallet, I'm convinced those girls spent more money on jeans, makeup, hair products, and parking tickets than the entire budget of the space project. As Kaitlyn was about to graduate from college, I calculated that it had cost over $230,000 to let that little breach-born-honeymoon-baby live upon the face of this earth. I'll admit that this fee included eighteen years of private education, but that price tag did not take into account her mother's personal birthing fees, pain and suffering, wear and tear, or bodily depreciation.

Of course there was the normal high school drama to contend with: best friends made and broken, boyfriends gained and lost. Then there were wardrobe malfunctions to be corrected, unruly eyebrows to be dealt with, the drama of "Proma" to be lived through, sisterly squabbles to mediate, and mani-pedi's to pay for. And let's not forget about those contentious curfews, concerts, and college applications. Is it any wonder that the brain of the woman who gave birth to these children was left spinning in a constant state of bewilderment?

I'd love to give you a scene from one of our home movies in those glorious days, but we appear to have stopped documenting our children's lives somewhere right around the time those girls entered their high school years. Coincidence? I think not. Never fear, for I have that blog which documented (with some exaggeration) the life of the poor motion-sick-mother instead:

> *The early morning mist had barely risen past the rim of her coffee cup as she paddled down the stairs in her home - each step less forgiving than the one before. An unknowing listener might think her stride light, but she alone knew just how heavy her heart had become. She was about to begin another day in a tedious life that sometimes pained one to live it; a life so dreary that even her wardrobe screamed to be released.*

*She approached the clothes dryer in search of her day's attire.
Once there, she methodically folded the palates of her everyday
existence - the blacks . . . the browns. . . the burgundies of her life
- when suddenly a strange light flashed through the material.*

*"Oh No!" cried she in dismay. "Don't tell me I ripped those
black pants again!"*

*But as she held the offending article up for inspection, she
discovered that those rays of light were not streaming through
unwanted openings. No, these holes were in a distinct and
beautiful pattern. It was lace! A texture memorable to her touch.
. . familiar to her skin . . . long ago forgotten.*

*How had this small piece of black lace wound its way through the
universe to become intertwined with her clothing? Had some
great cosmic static-cling storm caused it to land amid her
possessions? And, more importantly, what was the meaning
behind its arrival? Was it a portent sent to lift her from the
monotony of her life? To reinforce her solidarity with all of
womanhood?*

*And so she held that tangible sign of hope, caressing her cheek
with the subtle coarseness of the fabric, until. . .*

*Until she discovered a tag that read "Victoria's Secret"! This
wasn't merely a piece of lace. It was a* **THONG,** *and a size extra
small at that!!!!*

*Suddenly she was no longer wondering how that lace had found
its way into her clothes dryer. The only question remaining was,
"Which one of her teenage daughters had used that dryer before
she did?" For she knew with certainty that the contraband item
hadn't been spawned from her old-lady-granny-panties
overnight.*

And what should she do with this little (and I do mean little!)

piece of evidence? Confront her offspring? Show her husband? Dangle the offending article from the kitchen chandelier until the miscreant confessed? Or should she do nothing, waiting to see which one of her three daughters would begin to develop a look of utter desperation as Saturday night approached?

And then, quietly tucking the garment into her bathrobe pocket, she smiled and – for the first time in weeks – ascended the stairs with a spring in her step.

Yes those were the days my friends. And my daughters lived each one of them to their fullest. Thankfully only two – no maybe four – of their escapades involved encounters with the police. I really don't know whether to classify a one-night-two-daughter encounter with New York City EMS workers as a verifiable police experience or not.

I believe that I can confidently state that each of my girls entered their teenage years dancing over different hot coals, yet came through on the other side wiser, smarter, and more compassionate.

And me? I don't think that raising three teenage daughters is easy on any parent, but I'll admit right now, it was very rough for me. I worried like any other parent, and then worried like another ten parents combined. My daughters wanted to live a life like other healthy teenagers and yet I knew, deep down, that they were not healthy teenagers.

Worries, worries, worries.

Tumult, trials, and tears.

Letting Go

Letting my fledgling daughters fly from the nest was a big step for me. How would they survive their joint pain and fatigue without me there to fill their prescriptions? How would we manage doctor's appointments and labs? What if they got sick? I mean *really* sick.

Yet somehow despite it all I knew there would be a day in the future when I would have to let go, for there was the looming thought of college – a double edged sword in all honesty. In my heart of hearts I didn't want to let them go from under my watchful eye; yet my tired eyes could stand watching them no longer. For each of them, the time came when I was ready to let them go – although I'll admit that it became easier each time I waved goodbye.

For the most part, my fears went unrealized as we navigated though those years one step at a time. As I said, I was growing accustomed to living with uncertainty. That isn't to say that everything went smoothly during their time away at various universities. There were countless tough times and close calls. There was the night that Michael and I rushed from our home in New Jersey to a hospital in Connecticut because Raynaud's spasms in Kaitlyn's feet (called Raynaud's contractions which happen in response to cold) had become so concerning that the nurses in the college infirmary insisted she go to the local emergency room. We spent hours with her as they ran tests, warmed her feet until normal color returned, and then sent her back to her dorm room at 2:00 a.m.

As predicted, Megan also gave us a scare now and then. Can you imagine virtually talking your child through a visit to an emergency room in Virginia while you remain in New Jersey?

That happened numerous times with Megan as she was treated and sent back to her dorm with a diagnosis of dehydration, interstitial cystitis, or severe conjunctivitis.

Perhaps Leah's trip to the emergency room in Delaware one Sunday night was the most frightening of all, but we'll cover that in a later chapter.

Although the letting go part was hard at times, it was a gradual process, spurred on by positive outcomes and the absence of any real life-threatening events. I tried hard not to stifle my daughters' sense of adventure or let my own fears prevent them from doing things they wanted to do. Kaitlyn spent an entire semester in Florence and returned to travel in Europe immediately after her graduation. Leah traveled to Sweden and Spain during her junior year in college. They all went on volunteer trips to Appalachia with our church youth group, learning how to repair and rebuild houses. (Yes, someone was foolish enough to entrust those girls with a nail gun.) They traveled to Biloxi, Mississippi to provide help in the wake of Hurricane Katrina. Kaitlyn twice traveled to Guatemala to build homes for those without. Always the animal lover, Megan was able to fulfill her lifelong dream of swimming with the dolphins while on spring break in Florida.

Please allow me to relate a little story that I hope will help you to understand the process of letting go: When Megan was first diagnosed with her lupus-like illness, her rheumatologist stressed over and over again that she needed to stay out of the sun for two reasons: many lupus patients develop severe sun sensitivity; and one of the known causes of a lupus flare is sunburn.

We were a family who spent large portions of the summer at my parents' house at the "shore" (as we Jerseyites refer to what others call the "beach"). Going to the beach for hours on end was part of our lazy daily routine while we were seaside, and we would spend our afternoons at the local municipal swimming pool when we were at home. Megan particularly loved swimming in the ocean. She also had inherited her father's darker skin tone instead of her mother's fair Irish skin, and although I slathered sunscreen on her several times each day, she inevitably turned brown and tan each summer. It just happened.

When she was suddenly forbidden from spending time in the sun, it was the ultimate disappointment. My heart went out to her as we watched Kaitlyn and Leah, boogie boards in hand, skip off to the beach with my sister's family while we stayed back at the house. I tried my best to provide other entertainment for her. We watched movies, went shopping, or out to lunch. But in reality, nothing really replaces a day on the beach for a 12 year old. Her doctor was adamant and I was vigilant.

As the years went by and I began to lose both my influence and control over Megan's comings and goings, she began to insist upon going to the beach with her sisters. I, by this time, had developed a dislike of the sun and still opted to stay home, but I slowly let down my guard and did not stop her from going. Time proved that she was certainly not sensitive to the sun, and – just like when she was little – Megan's skin gradually tanned and never burned. She never suffered any ill effects from her time in the sun and I began to loosen my grip, and my fears, a little.

If that story didn't do it for you, let me try another one.

As I have already related, Kaitlyn spent a semester in Florence, Italy when she was a junior in college. Keep in mind that these were the days before the advent of international cell phones, so Michael made arrangements for her to rent a mobile phone while she was there. Aside from one brief email informing us that she had landed safely, two days into her journey, Michael and I had not heard from our eldest daughter. And so we eagerly awaited a call from her – for, of course, the act of paying for this cell phone did not include informing the parents of the actual phone number. Nor did it guarantee that the rentee would actually use that phone to call her parents. We did know, however, that the entire group was scheduled to spend that first weekend in Rome. So when the phone rang in our house at 8:00 p.m. on Saturday evening, a quick calculation of the time difference led me to the realization that it was 2:00 a.m. in Rome. Not the best time for a 20-year-old to be phoning her parents.

Although Michael was the one to answer the phone, I could hear the chaos in the background from across our living room. Female voices were frantically yelling as Michael queried into the phone, "Kaitlyn? Kaitlyn!"

Eventually she began to mumble something about a wallet, and Michael was then able to extract a muddled story about how her best friend's wallet had just been stolen by pickpockets. As he began to ascertain that Kaitlyn and her possessions were unharmed, police sirens started to fill the air and she quickly shouted, "I have to go now. I'll call you back later!"

And then there was dead air.

No caller I.D. back in those days. No FaceTime, texting, Instagram, or Snapchat. Just two worried parents who had no way of getting back in touch with their daughter who had been a witness to a crime in the early morning hours on the streets of Rome 4,280 miles away.

That, my friends, was I night that I really learned to let go.

I waited up for a few hours, proceeded to drink a few glasses of wine (because, God knows, I wasn't going to have to leave the house and pick her up somewhere) and when no call came, went to bed and speedily succumbed to the uninterrupted sleep of the dead.

The point of my story? Sometimes you are confronted with circumstances that are far beyond your reach, your influence, or your control. At times like this, worry is of no value. You quickly find that you have no choice but to trust that all will work out in the end.

And work out it did. Years later – in speaking about the incident – Kaitlyn admitted that she had also imbibed in a few too many alcoholic beverages that evening and had mistakenly dialed the only number she had programmed into that rental phone. Astute enough to realize that she didn't want to speak with her father in her current condition, she got off of that call as quickly as she could.

I'm not positive, but it's my guess that Kaitlyn was in no state to lose sleep over that phone call that night either.

6. Guillain-Barre Syndrome

Things may happen and often do
to people as brainy and footsy as you.

– Dr. Seuss

"That" Sick

I have alluded to Leah's additional illness and now you will get to hear her story.

As you know, Leah was diagnosed with arthritis when she was roughly 12 years old. It caused significant joint and muscle pain for her, but it was a rheumatic disease – not an autoimmune disease. For as much blood as she had drawn in the ensuing years, her ANA turned up positive a handful of times and eventually returned to normal levels. Not much attention was paid to it, for when one family member has elevated antibodies it is not unusual for another family member to be ANA positive, yet asymptomatic. Interestingly enough, one of those dreaded antiphospholipid antibodies also turned positive for a while and then went into hibernation again.

If I had to choose, I would have told you that Leah was the healthiest of our three daughters, for her arthritis rarely interfered with her activities. She led a healthy lifestyle, exercised often, and ate a nutrient-rich diet. In fact, there were months when Leah didn't even take her prescribed NSAIDs;

replacing them with herbal combinations which claimed to stop inflammation.

That little girl in the chiffon bathrobe had always been a go-getter, determined to live life to the fullest and come out on top. This tenacity served her well. She earned excellent grades in school, was a natural leader, had a bevy of close friends – not to mention that there had never been a shortage of young men knocking on our door.

When Leah started her last semester of her senior year in college, things changed drastically for her but I didn't quite catch on. As any mother of a college student will tell you, the preferred method of communicating with your daughter is through text messaging. If I tried to call her she was always in class, the library, out to dinner, or at a party. By the time she was free to speak with me, I would be long asleep in my bed. So, without the benefit of hearing her voice on the phone, I did not grasp the full force of what she was dealing with.

Her troubles had started during her fall semester as she became sick repeatedly with strep throat and bronchitis. (Yes, strep throat again!) In December, blood tests ordered by her rheumatologist showed elevated liver enzymes but an ultrasound showed nothing out of the ordinary so we decided to ride it out over the Christmas holidays. Sure enough, those levels returned to normal without any explanation.

A few days after she returned to school for spring semester, Leah came down with what we assumed was the flu. Upon recovering, she immediately was diagnosed with bronchitis again. I distinctly remember one text from her which read, "Mom, I'm dying here!" I wrote it off as a typical Leah overstatement; a danger when your sole means of communication is through texting.

We did talk eventually. I encouraged her to suck it up and attend class, worried that her last semester would get off to a bad start. She couldn't be *that* sick. Now could she?

She was. *That* sick.

The one thing I didn't take into consideration was that Leah was different when it came to being sick. She was the child who never wanted to admit she was down. Leah was the very child I dragged kicking and screaming into the ER with a case of appendicitis. In a cruel twist of fate, it turns out that I became ill at the same time. For the first time in my adult life, I came down with the flu and was out of commission for a full week and didn't have the energy or awareness needed to devote to her.

It all came to a head when Leah called one Sunday evening to tell me that she was running a fever of 102, had a terrible headache, and couldn't move her neck. None of her housemates were home and she was truly miserable. Fearing it was meningitis, I told her to call her best friend and ask her to come home and bring her to the emergency room immediately.

Leah's best friend was a godsend that night; calling and sending text messages with each test they ran. A spinal tap did not show the presence of any bacteria and so meningitis was ruled out. That same test did show an elevated presence of protein in her spinal fluid, but the doctors in the ER did not find that disturbing enough to warrant further investigation. They brought down her fever, gave her IV hydration, prescribed painkillers, and – like her sisters before her – sent her back home without any explanation of what was causing this.

Once I verified that Leah was still among the living the

following morning, the vertigo-challenged-anxiety-ridden-woman-who-gave-birth-to-her hopped into her car and drove to Delaware to pick her up and bring her straight to the rheumatologist's office in New York. There began a series of tests, labs, and doctors' visits that I still shudder to think about: CAT scans and MRIs of her back and neck; an additional visit to our local ER which included a MRI of her brain; a visit to a neurologist which initially turned up nothing unusual; and an appointment with an infectious disease doctor.

As these days and weeks unfolded, Leah began losing sensation in her left hand and then her feet. She developed muscle weakness in her legs and left arm. She was evaluated by a functional neurologist, who plainly saw that something needed to be done. An examination with a pain management doctor that very week revealed the same thing. You name it, that child was prodded, poked, and peeked at inside and out. Yet still no real answers.

And she was getting worse.

The pain in her back was increasing. At times her lungs hurt. Muscles in her legs and arms started twitching involuntarily. She ran a constant low-grade fever. And she slept all day, every day, on our family room couch with the dog right by her side. It somehow felt like a cruel "déjà vu" to me; bringing back memories of Megan's illness which remained unexplained for so long. Only this time we were dealing with specialists, not a pediatrician, and the tests and referrals were overseen by a top-notch rheumatologist. Where was the answer?

It became clear to us all that this was a neurological problem of some sort, and that we needed a second opinion from another neurologist. Luckily we were able to secure an appointment with a neurology group which was associated with yet-another premier hospital in New York City. We went for the first appointment on a Friday and were told to come back for an Electromyography (EMG) and nerve conduction study on Monday.

The results of these two tests showed what we already knew: Leah had loss of feeling and delayed response time in her feet, legs, arms, and hands. Combined with the finding of elevated protein in that initial spinal tap, this neurologist diagnosed her with a case of Guillain-Barre Syndrome (pronounced Ghee-yan Bah-ray.) Of course, Leah and I were not surprised with this whimsically named diagnosis because we had both explored every possibility and this was a disease that we had landed on time and time again, but my limited knowledge of Guillain-Barre Syndrome (GBS) had caused me to write it off. I thought that GBS moved rapidly through a person's body and attacked the lungs. I had heard horror stories about patients being placed on respirators and hospitalized for months. Although there may be a typical progression of symptoms of Guillain-Barre, not all patients present with the same symptoms at the same speed. The neurologist thought that Leah's case was comparatively mild and had already reached its peak. We had much to be thankful for. The damage had not reached her lungs and there was no need for hospitalization. She told us that, in time, Leah would recover on her own but prescribed some infusions to help speed her recovery.

At last, the mystery explained!

But GBS was also an autoimmune disease, and the more research I did, the more I discovered. And while I now know about GBS, there's a good chance you do not and so I will share with you some of the things I have learned.

As we have already seen, autoimmune reactions occur when the body's fighter cells somehow receive the wrong signals and turn on the organs or systems they were designed to protect. In Guillain-Barre Syndrome these fighter cells damage the covering or insulation of the body's major peripheral nerves (the myelin sheath) leading to numbness or weakness. The disease is characterized by the rapid onset of this numbness and paralysis of the legs, arms, breathing muscles, and face. The paralysis usually travels up the limbs from fingers and toes and is frequently accompanied by abnormal sensations, like numbness and tingling affecting both sides of the body.

The cause of GBS is unknown. About 50 percent of cases occur shortly after a viral or bacterial infection, some as simple and common as the flu or food poisoning.

The good news about Leah's diagnosis was that GBS is a relatively short-term disease and once the process stops, the sheath is able to regenerate. While there is no cure for GBS, treatment is aimed at reducing symptoms and speeding up recovery. The treatment that Leah's neurologist prescribed was a series of intravenous immunoglobulin (IvIG) infusions given at home by a visiting nurse. While each infusion made her feel weak and gave her flu-like symptoms, by the end of five sessions, she thought she was feeling some improvement. The rest of her recovery was left to time and Mother Nature.

The Aftermath

Recovery from GBS can range from six months to two years or longer. A particularly frustrating consequence of GBS is long-term recurrences of fatigue and exhaustion as well as pain and muscle aches. These can be aggravated by "normal activity" and can be alleviated by pacing activity and rest. The terms "pacing" and "rest" had never entered Leah's vocabulary before, much less been part of her plan of action. Once she began to feel somewhat better she tried to live life as she used to know it, but learned through a painful period of trial and error that there was a "new normal" she would have to adhere to.

I was heartbroken the weekend Leah went back to watch her friends graduate from college without her. Little did I know, but months previously I had paid (this, my friends, is why that child was nicknamed *Ponzi*) for her to go away on a post-graduation vacation. She went to that graduation prepared to accompany her friends but quickly decided that she could not keep up. No matter that the pace she failed to keep up here may have been as simple as overall beer consumption; it pained me to see Leah admit defeat and come back home.

A nearly identical process was repeated a few weekends that summer. Leah would go away for a weekend and return home on Sunday night completely wiped out from the activities of the weekend. She then would spend the next four days sleeping on the family room couch. At the end of that summer, Leah enrolled in two classes at our local county college and resolved to stay home and rest more often. Still, she somehow got ill and suffered a relapse. While she was able to successfully complete one of those two courses, she needed to withdraw from the other. Time. She still needed that precious time that a then-23-year-old did not want to give.

The holidays brought some strangely elevated liver enzymes and jaundice (remember she had experienced the exact same symptoms one year before – in advance of the onset of GBS?) and the New Year saw her still knocked down from her relapse. On a routine visit, the rheumatologist could not get standard reflex actions and so we returned again to the neurologist with the very big fear that her acute GBS had turned into the chronic form of the disease called CIDP.

A repeat of the nerve conduction study proved us wrong; showing no further damage to her nerve response time and so she was prescribed physical therapy and was sent home to wait it out. Again.

Leah's story is not yet finished. As I write this she still suffers from feelings of neuropathy, and new symptoms have appeared. We are waiting for a definitive diagnosis and I pray that the diagnosis, if it comes, does not add another chapter to this book.

7. Sjogren's Syndrome

I'm sorry to say so but, sadly it's true,
that bang-ups and hang-ups can happen to you.

– Dr. Seuss

I am sure you remember how, back in an earlier chapter I was
wringing my hands about all of the "whys" connected with
my family's illnesses.   The most often-thought why was
always the big one: *"Why can't this happen to me instead?"*
There is not a mother living who would not have begged for
the same thing in my shoes. No one ever wants to see her
children suffer and I would gladly have traded places with
them. I had my chance to be young and carefree. Every child
should. And so I wished that I could take their burdens from
them.

Love of Sickness

There was a point in my childhood when I might venture to
say that I enjoyed being sick.

I am the fifth of seven children which means my mother was
an extremely patient drill sergeant – raising a small army in
suburban New Jersey without the aid of cell phones,
voicemail, or even a second car. She gently cared for us when

we were sick, but had a sixth sense which allowed her to know when we were faking it. In order to stay home from school a child had to be verifiably ill, which meant vomiting or running a fever.

I never really warmed up to those stomach bug illnesses. Nor would I confess a fondness for my annual holiday throw-ups. (Yes, I could be counted on to – let's call it "upchuck" – on each and every holiday night, a combination of overeating and overexcitement.) Yet I could not help but enjoy the fever ills.

I loved the fact that my mother gave me special attention whenever I began to display anything more than an occasional sniffle. There was simply nothing better than spending the morning under the clean, crisp sheets she would insist on putting on my sickbed. I loved the feel of her practiced hand on my forehead and the icy-coldness of that mercury thermometer placed under my tongue. The wait to determine if that silver sludge had moved above the 98.6 mark was filled with hopeful anticipation, and the skillful way my mother shook that mercury back down again had me convinced she had foregone a job as conductor in a symphony orchestra just to tend to me. What's more, I cherished the taste of the baby aspirin which would follow. (Do not try this at home, folks, for those were days before we knew about mercury poisoning or the dangers of giving children aspirin.) Chicken noodle soup and its accompanying saltines arrived on a bed tray at lunchtime – the best room service any child could ask for.

Ice packs, hot water bottles, epsom salts, witch hazel – somehow, someway, my mother knew just what to do to make me feel better. And if my mother were to tell my father that I was *really* sick he would bring home flowers picked up in the train station on the way home from his job in New York City. That, my friends, meant that I had hit the jackpot.

This infatuation with being sick ended abruptly at age 11 when I was seriously ill for a full four days before my mother had the opportunity to take me to the emergency room. The better part of my precious summer vacation was then spent in the hospital with a ruptured appendix and ensuing peritonitis. My illness, although it passed my mother's verification test with both vomiting and fever, was ill-timed, for my mother was thrown out of her usual orbit. Through no fault of her own she was distracted – concerned with packing up from a family vacation, sending my older brother off to a new destination, attending a cousin's wedding, and hosting a barbeque on the Fourth of July.

Two major surgeries and five weeks later, I no longer had an interest in being sick. Those nurses and doctors did not care for me quite the way my mother did. I had to survive on a diet of ice chips for five days while a painful tube ran down my throat into my stomach. The thermometer I had so loved became my veritable enemy as it was placed in areas my mother had never attempted to approach since changing my diapers. That precious baby aspirin was replaced with countless bags of intravenous antibiotics. My life became a painful cycle of injections, infections, and irrigations. And no matter how many bunches of flowers I acquired from my father, I simply wanted to be home again. I will not go so far as to say that this appendectomy instilled an outright fear of the doctor, but I did develop a strong distaste for medical settings and institutional food.

Fear of the Doctor

Enough of this nostalgia; I intended to speak of current day maladies.

I will admit here and now that I acquired a significant case of anxiety while my daughters were going through their teenage years; any sane mother would have done so in my shoes. What you may not understand is that anxiety, by its very nature, is an insidious process. The fear crept up on me slowly day after day. And even when I recognized the fact that I had a problem, the overwhelming dread of doing the very thing which would help to alleviate it outweighed my concern about both my mental and physical health.

In order to fix the problem I needed to face my fear head on. I would have to pick up the phone and make an appointment. Not only that, I would have to drive to the doctor's office voluntarily and admit that I had let anxiety get the better of me. I just didn't have it in me.

What may seem even more incredulous to you is the fact that I was working full time and splendidly pretending to be a normal human being. I performed my job requirements exceptionally and was liked, praised, and admired by many. No one but Michael knew or would have guessed.

I won't bore you with the trivialities surrounding the major panic attack which blew my cover, but I finally made friends with an antidepressant/anti-anxiety medication and became even faster friends with an anti-anxiety medicine which I found useful for situational anxiety.

Yet when one develops Fear of the Doctor, (from here on, we'll refer to it by its acronym FOTD) it is not easily cured.

Although I was 50 years old and my mother was a breast cancer survivor, I had not had a mammogram in approximately five years. My father had contracted colon cancer at age 54, yet I had avoided having a colonoscopy. A phone call after my last visit to the gynecologist telling me that the results of my pap smear were irregular went unreturned. I had not visited the dermatologist despite the fact that my brother had melanoma and we shared the same Irish skin. I knew that at least one brother had been diagnosed with an autoimmune neuropathy, yet convinced myself that the numbness and tingling in my own feet were due to some sort of copycat syndrome. What's more, I changed dentists every two years due to the fact that – after having dental work done in one office – I could never bring myself to make another appointment.

It is a well known fact that FOTD can override both your common sense and your desire to be healthy. Yet there was one glimmer of hope; one tiny little thread. I had hypertension and knew that it would be irresponsible for me not to take a pill once a day to keep my blood pressure in check. Keeping on top of my blood pressure required quarterly trips to my primary care physician which I would invariably attempt to stretch out to semi-annual trips – for only after the doctor would refuse to refill my prescriptions would I reluctantly visit the office.

On one of these involuntary trips I got snagged for a full-blown physical, and since I was already exposed – paper gown and all – I asked my doctor to run an ANA blood test on me. I know it has been a while since I talked about an ANA, but it stands for anti-nuclear antibodies, a marker for some autoimmune diseases like lupus. I had suspected for some time that I may have been the source of my daughters' illnesses. I had recently turned 50 and knew that I was experiencing joint pain, especially in the morning, but what did I have to compare it to? How was a 50-year-old body supposed to feel? My husband had always been the model patient with the physique of an athlete. He ran, worked out, ate sensibly, took supplements, and did all of the things an individual should do to care for a body.

It was abundantly clear that his macaroni-and-cheese-loving-twice-baked-couch-potato wife could never compare herself to him.

When my ANA test came back abnormal my doctor referred me to the rheumatologist upstairs. At my first visit I was dismayed to see that the nurse who called me out of the waiting room was the mother of one of Leah's friends. What's worse, she insisted that my mac-and-cheese-loving-twice-baked-couch-potato body get on the scale so that she could weigh me.

Let me inform you now that if you are like me and have FOTD, you just may suffer from the further complication of DOTDS (Dread of The Doctor's Scale). Add to that the fact that you are actually acquainted with the person clinking that little weight from notch to notch, and the situation becomes intolerable. While I was quite positive that this particular nurse was a professional member of the medical community and would never go whispering my weight over her back fence, fear is fear, plain and simple.

In the interim, the rheumatologist did a physical exam, drew some blood, and told me to return in three weeks. Being the pragmatic individual that I am, I knew that the scale was never going to budge significantly in those three weeks, and so began to devise plans in order not to repeat the humiliation of that first visit. When the big day came, I used the tactic which I had used previously at my PCP's office and emphatically stated, "Oh, you just weighed me three weeks ago. No need to weigh me again!" To no avail. That professional nurse insisted that it was doctor's orders that I jump on that scale, and so I was forced to repeat the mortification of three weeks earlier.

Why do doctors still use those scales? Why do they not have a different, and more secretive, mechanism for weighing their victims? Why is it most often found in the common area? And did you ever notice how efficient those nurses appear once they have watched that little arrow bob up and down for an ungodly amount of time while your self respect hangs in the balance? Oh, they let it hover there like a beacon for any extra pounds looking for a home. But when they're finished? They close that thing down with a swooooosh faster than a French guillotine, leaving you to appear like nothing short of a slug as you attempt to creep off that wiggly instrument of torture.

And you wonder why I might have Dread of the Doctor's Scale?

The rest of the appointment was spent in a haze; for when one suffers from FOTD, complicated by DOTDS, one is not responsible for one's actions. And while I was sure my blood would test positive for the dreaded antiphospholipid antibodies, this rheumatologist told me it did not. What was positive was my anti-SS-A – a marker for Sjogren's Syndrome – a disease I had read about, but never considered before.

"Is that the one with the dry eyes and dry mouth?" I asked.

"Yes," he replied. He explained that the disease was an eponymous disease; named after a Swedish ophthalmologist named Henrik Sjogren who had first put the puzzle pieces together.

Even though the name of this strange sounding illness employed my beloved alliteration, I was not experiencing dry eyes or dry mouth and had no interest in being diagnosed with a disease I could not pronounce – much less one as boring and inglorious as that. I was adamant about not talking myself into a whole host of symptoms that didn't exist for me. So the visit ended in quite an undignified way, with me refusing treatment for Sjogren's Syndrome and promising to return in a year.

That was, until my DOTDS got in the way and I never set foot in that office again.

The Onset

The moral of my personal fairy tale is that you need to be specific when invoking the Wish Fairy. My hope was that I could somehow lift my daughters' burden off their shoulders and bear it instead of them, but somehow that silly fairy mixed up the "instead" part and added "also."

As mentioned in an earlier chapter, part of the reason why I was not on top of the onset of Leah's Guillain-Barre was the fact that I had come down with the flu myself a few weeks after she did.

I used to be one of those people who boasted that they never got sick. That's because – once I spent those five weeks in the hospital – I made it a point to never be sick again. If you seek proof, you can ask my husband. In the first 26 years of our marriage he had only seen me ill on one occasion. When the children were little and came down with stomach bugs I would sprint from room to room with the throw up bucket (as we lovingly called it) and never once caught the virus from them. I would nurse my tender offspring through countless fevers, fluxes, and flu's and never feel the ill-effects myself.

My sole weakness was my yearly cold. When I contracted a cold it would drop me to my knees. The most unbearable symptom was the constant stream of tears which would cascade from my eyes. Each eye would swell up as the virus moved from one side of my face to the other; leaving me looking like a prize fighter after a 12-round bout with a rhinovirus. In each of the two years previous to what I now view as the onset of Sjogren's Syndrome, I contracted my annual winter cold. Yet something was different with these two in that not a tear dropped from either eye. I thought to myself, "Aaaaah! This is what normal people feel like when they have a cold. It's so easy!"

Now back to my story.

I recovered from that flu slowly, but pushed myself to return to work as quickly as I could, for I had been out of the office on jury duty for eight days prior to getting sick and holy week was quickly approaching. After my daughters had grown I had taken a job as an administrator for a large Catholic church and the week between Palm Sunday and Easter was always a logistical nightmare for me. You might surmise that the job of being a "church lady" could not be stressful, but yet that week was for me. During this most sacred of marathons, the church building had to be decorated and re-decorated, configured and re-configured, no less than four times. There were countless liturgies to prepare, supplies to order, and participants to keep straight. I would arrive home each night smelling of incense, candles, and holy oils and pour myself into bed. Before I knew it, I was up pouring coffee into a to-go mug and heading off to work to repeat it all again.

That very week was also filled with physician appointments for Leah. She was scheduled for her nerve conduction study on Monday and an appointment with her rheumatologist on

Friday, both of which involved a trip to New York. I had also just received word that Megan's blood test results once-again showed a higher-level of disease markers which bumped my level of worry and anxiety up yet another two notches. How was I going to do all the work that needed to be done in the short amount of time I had? How would I oversee it all when I wouldn't even be in the same state at times? What would the results of Leah's testing show? And Megan, would she suffer a stroke or embolism at any moment?

I am unlike most of my fellow Sjogren's patients, in that I can clearly recall the day that I realized what was happening. Remember, I had the magical insight of knowing that I possessed the anti-SS-A antibody. Although I had shrugged it off, I suppose I never forgot because while at work on the Saturday immediately preceding Palm Sunday I suddenly felt my mouth dry up. Parched. Arid. Tongue strangely sticking to the roof of my mouth. Lips glued together. It was a sensation I had never experienced before.

I somehow made it through that holy, yet horrid, week. We received Leah's diagnosis of Guillain-Barre on Monday, confirmed by our trusty rheumatologist on Friday. Leah, herself, took the initiative in setting the wheels in motion to start the IvIG infusions. I simply didn't have the time. My two free hours on Holy Saturday (a 16 hour work day for me) were spent surreptitiously cleaning out my desk – preparing for what I knew I had to do. I was back at work by 8:00 on Easter morning and worked until 2:00 in the afternoon. As I left that day, I knew that I needed to take a leave of absence. I had other things to tend to.

Leah needed me. And I sensed what was happening in my own body and knew I needed me too.

Behind a Swedish Man's Name

It's time I told you a little more about this disease called Sjogren's (pronounced SHOW-GRINS) Syndrome.

Sjogren's is a disease like other autoimmune diseases in which the cells, normally called up by your body to fight infection, mistakenly begin to affect healthy cells instead. In the case of Sjogren's, these fighter cells target the moisture producing glands in your body – most specifically the glands which produce tears and saliva. The combination of the resulting dry eyes and dry mouth are commonly known as "sicca syndrome" (from the Latin *siccus*, meaning "dry").

Dryness inherent with Sjogren's can cause all sorts of problems. Chronic dry eye can cause corneal scratches, erosion, and decreased resistance to infection. Decreased saliva production can affect the ability to speak or taste and results in a significantly higher incidence of dental decay. With reduced saliva output, many Sjogren's patients develop swallowing difficulties and gastrointestinal reflux disease (GERD). As my dentist recently told me, her professor in dental school would often tell the class, "Saliva is a very expensive product."

The symptoms of Sjogren's may remain steady, worsen, or, uncommonly, go into remission. While some people experience only mild discomfort, others suffer debilitating symptoms that greatly impair their functioning. Severe joint pain and debilitating fatigue often accompany Sjogren's. Ninety percent of Sjogren's Syndrome sufferers are women. It is estimated that about half of Sjogren's patients have been diagnosed with the syndrome as their primary disease and the other half have it in conjunction with another disease such as thyroid disease, lupus, or rheumatoid arthritis.

Sjogren's, like lupus, is a systemic disease, which means it can affect other major organs in the body. Primary Sjogren's can affect lung, heart, liver, and kidney function. Nerves can develop carpal tunnel syndrome and peripheral neuropathy. Primary Sjogren's patients also have a higher risk of developing lymphoma.

Some people with Sjogren's Syndrome have certain autoantibodies circulating in their blood called "anti-SS A" and "anti-SS B" which are strongly, but not exclusively, associated with Sjogren's Syndrome. Other people with clear evidence of Sjogren's do not have those antibodies.

Currently there is no cure for Sjogren's Syndrome and treatment is mostly aimed at relieving symptoms. Although Sjogren's is one of the most prevalent autoimmune disorders, striking as many as four million Americans, it is one of the least studied and understood. In fact, there has not been one drug developed specifically to treat systemic Sjogren's. Yes, there are prescription drops for dry eyes and medications to increase saliva production, but all of the treatments used to treat extra-glandular complications have been borrowed from other diseases, most often lupus and rheumatoid arthritis. Drugs that suppress the immune system – in hopes of calming down the autoimmune response – are often used. Some of these are even low-dose chemotherapy drugs.

In many respects I am lucky; for I knew what was wrong with me and was spared the months (or more likely, years) of trying to piece together a group of disparate symptoms. The Sjogren's Syndrome Foundation estimates that the average time from onset of symptoms to diagnosis is more than three years. Can you even imagine?

During the course of that horrific – I mean holy – week I had the presence of mind to call and make an appointment with another rheumatologist (with an unknown nurse to weigh me, mind you.) I had to wait approximately one month for my first appointment, where – based on my symptoms and positive SS-A marker – she made a definitive diagnosis of primary Sjogren's Syndrome and sent me off for a round of testing with other specialists, including a hematologist to follow-up on what were now my positive antiphospholipid antibodies.

By this time, fatigue and joint pain had set in and I had all I could do to drag myself from one doctor's appointment to the next. For if, perchance, you thought I had become somewhat undone in my previous years raising my daughters, I need not tell you what it is like to have my life completely unravel after being diagnosed with an autoimmune disease of my own.

For someone who spent much of her adult life avoiding doctors at all costs, I dare say there isn't an "ologist" I haven't visited since being diagnosed. I started, as you know, with the rheumatologist and moved quickly through the optometrist, ophthalmologist, hematologist, pulmonologist, dermatologist, psychiatrist, gastroenterologist, podiatrist, and neurologist.

As if the "ologists" weren't enough, I've also had to contend with the "itis" business. Since being diagnosed, I have been treated for diverticulitis, gastritis, esophagitis, duodenitis, tendonitis, and neuritis. Add to that impingement, radiculopathy, neuropathy, corneal abrasions and erosion, swollen salivary glands, carpal tunnel syndrome, and GERD. And let us not forget an essential tremor which makes my hands shake and an esophageal motility disorder which means I often can not swallow pills or food without feeling them lodged in my throat.

A full 13 vials of blood were taken at my first appointment with the rheumatologist and countless needles have found their way in to draw out my precious lifeblood since.

I have undergone three chest X-rays to rule out lymphoma (where they snagged me for that long overdue mammogram) tear production and break-up tests, four nerve conduction studies, three abdominal CT scans, an endoscopy (along with that other dreaded "oscopy" that only old people talk about), an at-home sleep study, pulmonary function testing, an echocardiogram, cortisone shots, two MRIs of my brain, an MRA of my head, and X-rays and MRI of my feet and ankles. I have spent weeks in physical therapy strapped into a machine stretching calf muscles which never bothered me and providing therapy for a pinched sciatic nerve which caused me no pain. And let us not forget the multiple trips to the dentist for an extraction, root canals, crowns, extra cleanings, and fillings.

I now take prescription medication for acid reflux, joint pain, nerve pain, inflammation, an immunosuppressant anti-rheumatic, and the same anti-malarial medication which was first prescribed for Megan. Add those to the four medications I was already taking on a regular basis and you get a total of ten medications – and 15 pills – I need to manage each day. I also use a combination of five different eye drops to deal with my eye symptoms.

The anti-malarial drug, plaquenil, has been found to relieve some of the underlying fatigue and pain associated with lupus and rheumatoid arthritis, but does not appear to be as effective in Sjogren's patients. As we found out with Megan it takes six months to feel its full effects, and by that stage of my illness my symptoms had gotten worse, not better. I continue to take it twice a day, however, for I'll never know if it's alleviated some of the fatigue. Sometimes you simply can't prove a negative.

Plaquenil is just one of a class of medications typed as Disease Modifying Anti-Rheumatic Drugs (DMARDs.) Other medication in this class of drugs are low-dose version of a chemotherapy drugs meant to calm the immune system. These immunosuppressants are intended to alleviate the process which causes inflammation; relieving joint and muscle pain and halting the progress of the disease. And while it seems we can't turn on the television these days without viewing advertisements for new "biologic" drugs used to treat rheumatoid or psoriatic arthritis, these drugs routinely have not been tested on Sjogren's patients and so are not approved by Medicare or private insurance companies.

My Daily Bread

When I originally left my job at the church it was on a three month family leave in order to nurse Leah back to health. As the weeks crept by and she started to experience the benefits of the infusions, Leah's symptoms started waning while my own began waxing.

I had promised to return to work at the beginning of August, yet I quickly realized that I could not return to my old level of activity. There was no question about it; my body would not allow me to do it. I felt quite sure that – even if my responsibilities were reduced enough to allow me to work part-time – I would not be able to keep up. My dry eyes could not stare at a computer screen all day. Nor could my arthritic-ridden and tremor-laden fingers type on its keyboard or spend any amount of time writing longhand. What's more, the arid environment in my mouth prevented me from having long phone conversations. And the fatigue? The crushing sensation of fatigue was the overriding factor that made the thought of returning to work a non-starter.

As time slipped by, I grew more and more anxious about returning to work. I knew in my heart of hearts that I could never handle those demanding hours of work again, and every time I thought about it, it brought back flashbacks of a different time. . . a different me . . . a me that I instinctively knew would never be again. My husband and my rheumatologist both understood and agreed. And so my family leave became a disability leave.

I know you have heard the term "Catholic guilt" before, but just imagine what it feels like to walk away from a job where God is your boss.

In retrospect I realize that, although I really didn't want or mean to quit God, I needed to let go of some things I thought I was doing in his name but was perhaps doing for my own reasons. I needed to stop trying to be superwoman in other's eyes. I needed to stop pretending I was strong. And perhaps I needed to be a little less of a control freak. I always said that if I were God, I would like a clean church. Why else would they say that cleanliness was next to Godliness?

But I was not a prophetess, spokeswoman, or housekeeper for God, now was I? No, I was simply a person who needed to let God be God without trying to act as his personal assistant. It is a very painful lesson for someone like me to learn that God is the one who is the architect of the plans for my life, and *that* thought had to come crashing down on my head in order for me to take note. Instead I waited for the train wreck to hit. And hit it did. So now I can't go up or down a flight of stairs without pain. I cannot walk through a grocery store without feeling fatigue. And I cannot eat a mere cracker without liquid with which to wash it down.

As if I needed yet another reason to be thankful that God invented wine!

8. Both Sides Now

Why fit in when you were born to stand out?
– Dr. Seuss

Terrible Two's

It may be nothing more than a wild hunch, but I have decided that my family's bad luck may come in twos.

It is a proven fact that my children have clearly had the tendency to come down with illnesses at the same time – be it chicken pox, colds, or stomach bugs. One summer Kaitlyn broke her right arm falling down the stairs and her left arm tripping on the boardwalk. Megan visited the emergency room exactly one year to the day after a previous year's visit. On another occasion, Leah occupied the same bay in the ER two days in a row. My mother and I were both assigned the exact same bed in a 702 bed hospital, only six months apart.

Perhaps the craziest story is the one, years ago, when Leah and Megan – young and seemingly carefree teens – were rushed via ambulance to the same emergency room from a concert in New York City within an hour of each other. (As to what precipitated these visits, let me advise any interested readers that when raising red-blooded American teenagers, keeping inventory of your household vodka bottles is always a good idea – for they both suddenly came down with an *Absolut*-ly dreadful sickness of mysterious origins.)

There are no words to describe the way a mother feels when walking into an emergency room and seeing two of her daughters lying on gurneys next to each other. And just like those times when they were younger and I would sprint from room to room with our infamous throw up bucket, Kaitlyn and I spent a long night holding those little hospital basins while my other daughters emptied the contents of my liquor cabinet into them. (Luckily for the two culprits, the husband of the household just happened to be out of town on a business trip.)

Did I relate this story just to embarrass them? Perhaps, but I also told it to demonstrate how I felt trying to manage Leah's illness while growing sicker myself each day.

I didn't know how to help us both.

Leah took up residence on the family room couch, while I claimed the couch in the living room. We both spent (and continue to do at times) a good part of the day napping on our respective couches. When the visiting nurse came to administer Leah's infusions I forced myself to run an errand or two. If I somehow mustered the energy to do the grocery shopping, I would often falter when it was time to prepare the food.

While the hallmark symptoms of Sjogren's hit me with a bang, some of the other, extraglandular problems crept up on me more slowly over the course of the summer and fall. Try as I might, I continued to get worse instead of better.

Was I devoting enough time to helping Leah? Was I still being a good mother? A loving wife? Responsible daughter?

And who was there to mother me?

Was this the level of pain and fatigue my daughters had been experiencing all along? Did they feel isolated like I did? Did they look at their healthy peers and friends and bemoan their own fate? Was this lonely, crappy feeling a staple in their lives too? This was taking empathy to a whole new level!

And sometimes a girl just can't help herself. Somehow you get sucked into the *"My pain is worse than your pain"* debate. By this time, Kaitlyn had long moved out of the house, but Megan had moved back in after graduating from college. When I would complain about my knees or ankles hurting Megan would quip, "I know Mom. I live with it every day!" When I suddenly made groaning noises going up and down the stairs, I would spy my two younger daughters rolling their eyes. My children had all lived with their pain so long they couldn't remember what it was like to live without it. I could.

To this day, when it's time to do simple chores like emptying the dishwasher or getting up to feed the dog, we still sometimes point at each other, claiming that we can't possibly be the one to hobble over there and do it.

But I'm their mother!

Years ago my mother could fix my ills with baby aspirin and witch hazel. I can't do that. I can only try to give them the support they need and remember to tell them every once in a while that I am in awe of how they have been able to deal with the challenges fate has thrown their way.

Shared Sisterhood

If there is one positive thing that my daughters' shared illnesses has done, it has been to bond them as sisters through a collective experience. These girls are not alone in this world – they belong to their own secret sorority (Ξ Felta Crappy Too.) Even if at times pain prevents one or another of them from performing the secret handshake, it is their heart embrace that really matters.

Kaitlyn, as the oldest, has led by example. She, in many ways, has perfected the art of being an eldest child. She serves as model and mentor, confidante and cheerleader. There isn't a medication or symptom she has not made herself familiar with. She is a proponent of a healthy diet and exercise, and always makes herself available when her sisters come to her with questions and problems. I dare say she now stands in for me on occasion. When she was young, members of the extended family used to call Kaitlyn the "pivotal cousin" because of her knack for making each person feel as if they are the center of her world. Her smile and enthusiasm are contagious; leaving the rest of us mere humans no choice but to want to be part of her circle.

Megan chose her undergraduate major in psychology well. While Megan is certainly more pensive than either of her other sisters, she is the one you trudge to with your troubles. Yes, she may be the only child in the history of mankind to return a purchase to a dollar store, but that is because she takes great care in making decisions. Megan also possesses a magical insight into the way the rest of us think and behave. She is, above all else, generous to a fault. If my three daughters were deserted on an island, Megan would give her sisters the last of her pain meds. And that, my friends, is munificence in motion.

Let us just take that example a bit further. If, as stated above, my three daughters found themselves on an island by themselves, Kaitlyn would be the one to make sure that they each had shelter and food. Megan would tend to their emotional needs and then run off to spend hours in the forest foraging for the right regalia for them to wear. And Leah? Leah, in all likelihood, would be the one to devise a way off of that island.

Please permit me to relate just one more of my favorite family memories captured on home video:

> The scene takes place in the family teepee the very day that Kaitlyn has returned home from the third grade class trip to the Native American cultural grounds. All three offspring have made an attempt to array themselves in native attire. The regalia of the newly-appointed tribal chieftess, has been purchased with wampum sent on that expedition for souvenirs. Megan's ceremonial dress has come straight from the basement box labeled "Halloween Costumes." Forced to be content with her sisters' cast-offs, Leah has attired herself in a grass hula skirt and pink cowgirl vest.

> The Chieftess leads her two squaw sisters in a traditional rain dance around the family room coffee table. The whoops and woo's can be heard; steps and skips clearly seen. The tribal elders are filled with assurance that umbrellas will be employed on the street at any moment.

> Suddenly the youngest squaw can be seen breaking from the circle and approaching the camera. She peers directly into that lens and whispers, hand at mouth, "This is re-dic-li-ous!" Once her views are on record, she rejoins her

sister warriors and continues with their traditional dance, proving the old Cheyenne proverb, "If a man is as wise as a serpent, he can afford to be as harmless as a dove."

Now that I have joined their ranks, I am not quite sure that my daughters' bond has extended to include me as a full member of their tribe, but I don't mind that. The important thing is that my own illness has given me a greater respect for my daughters.

Little House of Illness

I have wrestled with this idea for a number of months now. Could I be fostering a culture of sickness in our household? Have we somehow started to feed off each other's illnesses? Bodies of menstruating females living together often align in their hormonal cycles. Could the same thing be happening in our household? Within three days of arriving in our domicile our poor little cat Giardia Jax was back at the vet, ill with a fever.

And what about the factitious disorder, Munchausen Syndrome? Or – worse still – Munchausen Syndrome by Proxy? Both disorders are marked by attention-seeking behaviors centered on the health of yourself or your child. Is it possible that I am making this up? Could I be taking mild, benign disorders and spinning them into life-altering illnesses? Might I be creating a new disease called *Wilkey Syndrome?*

Why would I even be wondering about acquiring yet-another eponymous and crazy (and I do mean crazy) syndrome when

I have enough to worry about? Let's face it, I may be whacky and just a wee bit zany, but I have empirical evidence to confirm the existence of my disease. As do my daughters. If you seek proof of the depths of my symptoms, please visit my dentist. She's thrilled when I walk through the door, for not only do I always need dental work, she claims that I am her model patient (I am her *only* Sjogren's patient) and that other dentists can only drool over the thought of a completely dry environment in which to do their dastardly drilling.

Yet still I worry about setting the right example for my daughters. I wonder if surrendering so quickly to my disease was the right thing to do. Should I have tried to tough it out longer? Isn't it the Momma Bear's job to be strong and healthy in order to nurse her young cubs back to health? How can they expect to recover themselves when their mother's pill case is bigger than most mothers' handbags?

Do I cling to my disease? Use it as a crutch? Some people are known to wear their ailment like a warm, cozy sweater and grow so comfortable in it that they are afraid to take it off. Every chronically ill person should, at one time or another, stop and ask themselves, "Do I wish to be well again?" In some cases, our answers may surprise us.

But there's another side of the coin for me to consider. My situation is unique in that my first thoughts always go to my daughters. How, in heaven's name, could I wish, hope, or pray myself cured while my children remain sick? Hence, the mere fact that I know my daughters also suffer grounds me in a way that nothing else could. And if, by chance, my unbounded fantasies stray so far as to include a release from my illness, these thoughts are cut off mid-stream. No prayer, no wish, and no aspiration will be allowed to find me first in line to reap the benefits.

9. Peripheral Neuropathies

In the house, and on the street
how many, many feet you meet.

— Dr. Seuss

After regaling you with a bevy of heartfelt and wacky stories regarding my daughters, I feel compelled to warn you ahead of time that this particular chapter may prove to be slightly off-putting for even the most adventurous reader. The bright side is that it has plenty of big, important sounding words which offer the opportunity to improve your vocabulary.

The down side is that it is almost entirely about feet.

Not only is the subject of this chapter feet, it revolves around my brothers' feet (note that the plural means two siblings; four feet in total) along with my own, because each of us have a different autoimmune-mediated peripheral neuropathy.

Although many may have since followed in my footsteps, I firmly believe that I can claim the rights to being the original Seussophile. And Theodor Seuss Geisel may just be the only poet on earth who can claim the rights to creating an ode to the perambulating appendage, naming it, *"The Foot Book"*.

Because Dr. Seuss was not an actual physician, I often wonder if he was aware of the fact that there are 26 bones in the human foot, along with 33 joints, 107 ligaments, and 19 muscles and tendons. Did you know that the 52 bones in your feet make up about 25 percent of all the bones in your body?

Add to this the myriad of nerve branches which terminate in the feet and I believe that Leonardo da Vinci was correct when he stated that "The human foot is a masterpiece of engineering".

But did you ever think about how those 66 combined joints can cause a heck of a lot of pain when inflamed? About the tenderness that arrives when things go awry with those muscles and tendons? The strange combination of numbness and pain associated when those nerves run out of kilter?

The Neuropathy Association estimates that over two million Americans suffer from peripheral neuropathies. Peripheral neuropathy is the term used to describe disorders resulting from injury to the peripheral nerves. The term "peripheral" refers to anything outside of the brain and spinal cord. The peripheral nervous system contains the nerves that connect the central nervous system to the muscles, skin, and internal organs. The nerves themselves carry information from one part of the body to another. The axon is the part of the nerve that carries these impulses. Many of these axons are wrapped with a protective insulation called the myelin sheath. Those that are wrapped in this sheath are large fibers. Hence, when troubles arise in these nerves, either in the myelin sheath or the axon itself, it is called "large fiber neuropathy." Conversely, when smaller nerves no longer wrapped in the myelin sheath, are affected it is referred to as "small fiber neuropathy."

There are many types of peripheral neuropathies, only a few of which are autoimmune in nature. Neuropathy can be caused by diseases that affect only the peripheral nerves or by conditions that affect other parts of the body as well. For instance, it can occur as a result of chemotherapy treatment, or appear along with diseases such as diabetes. Symptoms almost always involve weakness, numbness, or pain – usually in the arms and legs.

Chronic Inflammatory Demyelinating Polyneuropathy

One of the autoimmune-related neuropathies is Guillain-Barre Syndrome (GBS) which we have already learned about. Another is Chronic Inflammatory Demyelinating Polyneuropathy (CIDP). In both diseases the neuropathy is caused when the immune system mistakenly destroys the myelin sheath of nerves. The end result is the loss of feeling in the area affected – most often starting with the feet and ascending upwards from there. As if the loss of feeling and motor control isn't enough, this type of large fiber neuropathy is often accompanied by a strange combination of numbness, tingling, pain, and weakness. If the reaction is able to be stopped the myelin sheath will regenerate, but with CIDP the disease progresses either with repeated attacks or in a steady fashion.

If you remember the process that was happening to Leah's nerves in her bout with GBS, it is easy to understand CIDP. It turns out that Guillain-Barre is simply (I don't mean simply, really, more like simply as in "boiled down to") the acute version of the very same autoimmune disease with which my oldest brother has been diagnosed. As with other autoimmune diseases, the reaction is thought to be triggered by an infection. In my brother's case, he started noticing his symptoms after a bout of influenza.

There is no cure for CIDP and treatment is aimed at slowing or halting the progression of nerve damage. My brother's physician has prescribed IvIG (Intravenous Immunoglobulin) infusions which he has been undergoing on a monthly basis for over 18 years – the very same infusions Leah received in more rapid succession when first diagnosed with GBS.

So the exact same process in my oldest brother's long-term neuropathy was what was happening in Leah's acute syndrome. The myelin sheath surrounding her nerves was being damaged through an autoimmune process – only with GBS the damage was happening at a rapid pace – causing her to leapfrog my brother in severity of symptoms.

Two feet down; four to go.

Axonal Neuropathy

If you thought wrapping your brain around the phrase, Chronic Inflammatory Demyelinating Polyneuropathy is difficult, imagine having to admit being diagnosed with a condition ingloriously named a Monoclonal Gammopathy of Undetermined Significance (or the equally ugly sounding acronym, MGUS)

Another one of my brothers not only has to pronounce it – he has to live with it.

And this MGUS has brought with it another type of nerve disorder; an autoimmune neuropathy where the axon itself is being damaged. The axon is the part of a nerve that carries impulses. This axonal neuropathy presents itself with progressive loss of sensation, pain, and weakness as the axon which carries the nerve impulses throughout the body degenerates. This neuropathy does not discriminate. These nerves can be the larger, myelin-covered motor or sensory nerves. They can also be smaller, fiber sensory nerves as well. Once again, there is no cure and treatment is aimed at relieving the pain.

Some may say that it is mere coincidence that two brothers have acquired two separate and distinct neuropathies in their adult years. Added to the rest of what I now know, I would proclaim that it is no coincidence.

Neuropathy Associated with Sjogren's

Peripheral neuropathy is a common complication in those with Sjogren's Syndrome. The causal relationship is not clear. Understood or not, the end result is that the sensory capacity in my own feet has become jumbled; causing my feet to feel painful, numb, and dead, all at the same time. I do not pretend to know, or compare, my feeling (or lack of it) with my brothers' and daughter's neuropathies. Nor will I tell you about their respective winding roads to their separate diagnoses. I will only bore you with my own.

While my feet silently feel numb, asleep, and crowded throughout the day, at some point during the night they start to scream. This lone symptom began long before my dry eyes and dry mouth. It began with a throbbing in my toes during the night a few years back which hurt so that I needed to keep my feet outside of the bedclothes because something as simple as a sheet resting on my toes would be excruciating painful. I have since read that neurological complaints often precede the dry eyes and dry mouth of Sjogren's. Perhaps if I had known this I would have paid more attention to the rheumatologist and his instrument of weight torture all those years ago.

Not long after being diagnosed with Sjogren's, an EMG and nerve conduction study was performed at my local hospital, revealing no delay time or lack of response. No surprise there. Sjogren's often targets nerves which are not tested on a normal nerve conduction test. Typical nerve-conduction tests are only sensitive to damage in the large-fiber nerves and do not detect abnormalities in the smallest-caliber nerves. A skin biopsy is the only way to assess the damage to small fibers common in Sjogren's patients and those biopsies should be performed in one of several highly reliable labs. The decision was made not to perform a biopsy, but to prescribe medication to relieve nerve pain nevertheless.

It was unclear to me whether I was dealing with one or two separate issues. I was also experiencing the spreading and splaying of my toes; for the piggy who ate roast beef began to pull apart from the piggy who stayed home – causing each of those last three toes to perform a crazy mixed-up dance, and resulting in a toe-traffic-jam of enormous proportions. In fact, the discomfort is such that *all* of my piggies detest going to the market and yearn to stay home instead.

But dealing with my foot problems was nothing to laugh about and the doctors' diagnosis's proved to be a bit ticklish. After three podiatrists, two neurologists, one foot and ankle specialist, three sets of x-rays, three nerve conduction studies, two rounds of physical therapy, and one MRI, I still had no definitive answer.

Eventually I had those biopsies for small fiber neuropathy performed. These biopsies confirmed that the number of functional small fiber nerves near my ankles and knees have been markedly reduced and those further up my thigh are already showing signs of deterioration. A final nerve conduction study revealed that I also have developed some large fiber neuropathy as well, causing my latest neurologist to order monthly infusions of Intravenous Immonoglobulin (IvIG) to try to slow, or perhaps halt, the progression of my neuropathy.

Carpal Tunnel Syndrome

Carpal tunnel syndrome is a common neuropathy in which the body's nerves become entrapped, compressed, or damaged. The carpal tunnel is a small narrow pathway in the wrist comprised of ligament, bones, and the body's median nerve which runs from the forearm, through the wrist, and into the palm and first four fingers of the hand. Sometimes thickening of the tendons or other swelling can press on the nerve, causing it to become compressed or entrapped. The result is numbness, tingling, pain, and loss of grip strength.

Carpal tunnel syndrome is another neuropathy which often accompanies Sjogren's Syndrome and is most likely due to generalized inflammation inherent with the disease. I have dealt with the effects of carpal tunnel syndrome for a while now, but chocked my symptoms up to something akin to the neuropathy in my feet. It started when my hands began to fall asleep numerous times throughout the night. This "paresthesia" then began to extend into the daylight hours as I drank my morning coffee, spoke on the telephone, or used my iPad. The neurologist prescribed splints for me to wear on both wrists at night. In time, excruciating pain arrived in my wrist, arm, and shoulder at night. The appearance of this pain at various times throughout the day became the catalyst for a return trip to the neurologist, a nerve conduction study on my arms, and the diagnosis of carpal tunnel syndrome in both wrists. This, in turn, resulted in another round of oral prednisone and cortisone shots to try and reduce the inflammation in my wrists.

When conservative measures such as splints, anti-inflammatory medicines, and cortisone shots don't work, surgery to cut the carpal ligament and relieve the compression is often performed. This is not an ideal means to get to a much longed-for end, but at least I know that I have the option of ridding myself of just one of my disparate symptoms for good.

10. A Diagnostic Tangle

Everything stinks till it's finished.

– Dr. Seuss

We now return to Leah and the fact that, 18 months after her diagnosis of Guillain-Barre Syndrome, she was still experiencing leg and back pain along with some new, unsettling symptoms. Her vision became blurry at times. Her heart rate was elevated while standing. Her muscles developed tremors, twitches, and cramps. She even exhibited some temporary gait problems.

Needless to say, we all became concerned. As stated in the preface to this book, the biggest risk factor in developing any one autoimmune disease is the fact that you have been diagnosed with another.

By this time Leah was working with a specialized physical therapist who was appalled at her condition. Disappointed with the wait-it-out approach prescribed by her neurologist in New York and worried that it had somehow spread to her central nervous system, we made an appointment with yet-another neurologist nearby. Admittedly he ordered all of the right tests for Leah. She had further MRIs on her brain and cervical, thoracic, and lumbar spine to rule out our collective fear of Multiple Sclerosis. The blood work he ran for evidence of other neurological causes of her problems proved to be negative. Her nerve conduction study and EMG revealed only slight irregularities which caused him to diagnose her with pinched nerves in her cervical and lumbar spine. He then suggested shots in her spine to relieve her pain.

More than a bit skeptical of his diagnosis (remember re-dic-li-ous?) we then visited a neurosurgeon who sat with us and reviewed her MRIs, proving vertebrae by vertebrae, how Leah's nerve openings were sufficiently open and certainly not pinched.

Could it be that she was still suffering from the residuals of her bout with Guillain-Barre?

There was still so much that did not make sense. Besides the pinched nerve already mentioned, Leah collected a myriad of different diagnoses (some correct, and many not so. . .) during this prolonged recovery from GBS. These diagnoses ran the gambit from hives to Hashimoto's, Crohn's to cystitis, Addison's, asthma, and allergies. I don't think I have the words to describe the agony I feel for Leah, trapped in an endless round of doctor's appointments, tests, and varied, conflicting, and often-incorrect diagnoses. While she was pro-active in trying to resolve her illness for the better part of two years, I began to sense a bit of apathy creeping in. Who could blame her?

What happened to that spunky little girl who screamed at the attendant to release her from the Froggy Ride? The three-year-old determined to beat her older sisters in the Easter egg hunt? Where was that tenacious young girl who danced in the school talent show just four days after having her appendix removed?

Trapped in the lethargic web of chronic illness is my guess.

And as for the woman who had the honor of being her mother? Imagine my dismay and worry as I placed my faith in each of these diagnoses. If you believed each one, as I tended to do, I had given birth to a child who was missing sensation over a large part of her body and whose connective tissues had somehow become undifferentiated. Not only that, but she was fighting endometriosis and an irritated, overactive bladder, while unable to control her involuntary nervous system. About to go into an adrenal crisis at any moment, the same poor soul was suffering from Crohn's disease, and pernicious anemia, asthma, Hashimoto's Thyroiditis, two pinched nerves, cysts on her spleen and ovaries, jaundice from a benign disease called Gilbert's Syndrome, and hives all over her body to boot!

I became so immersed in Leah's condition, I believe that I may now know more about the workings of the human body than most medical students. They can have the pleasure of working on their cadaver as part of their anatomy lab, I'll stick with the bone-of-my-bone and flesh-of-my-flesh patient.

From within the tangle of this diagnostic nightmare, Leah somehow picked up the threads of three autoimmune diseases which turned out to be the most important: thyroid disease, vitamin B12 deficiency, and undifferentiated connective tissue disease. I will give you a brief overview of these three.

Hashimoto's Disease

It will be no surprise to learn that in Hashimoto's Thyroiditis the immune system attacks and destroys the thyroid gland. The thyroid then produces too little hormone and the body's metabolism slows down. It is the most common of all the thyroid conditions and women are affected ten times more often than men. Symptoms, which often develop gradually, include fatigue, increased sensitivity to cold, dry skin, puffy face, hoarse voice, weight gain, joint pain, and muscle weakness. There is, once again, no cure for thyroid disease but synthetic hormones are used to replace those which are normally secreted by the thyroid gland. Getting the correct levels of these hormones is a balancing act for most patients, and any change in dosage takes weeks (or sometimes months) to take effect.

Pernicious Anemia

Pernicious anemia occurs when the intestines cannot properly absorb vitamin B12. The body needs this vitamin to make red blood cells. A protein called intrinsic factor helps your intestines absorb vitamin B12. In pernicious anemia, the body's immune system attacks the actual intrinsic factor or the cells in the lining of your stomach that make it. Symptoms can include fatigue, shortness of breath, dizziness, yellowish skin, irregular heartbeat, numbness or tingling, muscle weakness, and mental confusion. Nerve damage can be permanent if treatment does not start within six months of symptoms. There is no cure, and – in the past – pernicious anemia was a deadly disease, but now physicians can provide the needed B12 by injecting it intramuscularly; bypassing the need for the missing intrinsic factors.

The National Institute of Health reports that patients with Hashimoto's disease have an increased incidence of pernicious anemia, suggesting that the two diseases have a close relationship.

Undifferentiated Connective Tissue Disease

Remember how we talked about how Megan's second rheumatologist rescinded the first's diagnosis of lupus? We also talked at the time about how hard these types of diseases are to nail down because so many of them share symptoms and sometimes even test results. Undifferentiated connective tissue disease (UCTD) is another autoimmune disease that is used to describe people who have the symptoms and test results of a particular autoimmune disorder, but not enough of them (or just the right kind) to be fully classified by diagnostic criteria. Instead they seem to have a similar disorder that doctors call undifferentiated connective tissue disease. Although the word "undifferentiated" sounds vague, rheumatologists know this term describes a real problem. Over time, people with UCTD may evolve into one of the more specific connective tissue diseases, such as lupus, Sjogren's or scleroderma.

In Leah's case we know that she is leaning towards a "pre-lupus" type of diagnosis. Much, in fact, like her sister Megan. But Leah has two other autoimmune conditions with which to contend. As to the myriad of other autoimmune-related conditions that still may be lurking, we once-again are in a "wait and see" mode.

11. Multiple Autoimmune Syndrome

And Sally and I did not know what to do.
So we had to shake hands with Thing One and Thing Two.
We shook their two hands, but our fish said, "No! No!
Those things should not be in this house! Make them go!"
— *Dr. Seuss*

I bet we all wish that our story were over by now. No one wishes it more than I.

Approximately 25 percent of patients with one autoimmune disease have a tendency to develop another. The presence of at least three autoimmune diseases in the same patient has been defined as multiple autoimmune syndrome. As we can see, Leah fits this classification. I have recently learned that I may too.

A Bump in the Road

In our chapter on Sjogren's Syndrome I stated that approximately half of the time Sjogren's is the primary (only) disease acquired and the rest of the time it comes in conjunction with diseases such as lupus, rheumatoid arthritis, or thyroid disease. When first diagnosed, I had no signs of any other disease process in my body. My worst complications have always tended to be neurological in nature. Beyond the first-line treatment of plaquenil and steroids (which are used sparingly) the treatment protocol for more advanced or troublesome Sjogren's is to work through a series of disease modifying anti-rheumatic drugs (DMARDs) in hopes that one will work to relieve joint pain and fatigue and halt or slow the progress of the disease.

I had worked my way through two of these medications over the course of about nine months and discontinued them each because of side effects. I was also dealing with what I knew was worsening neuropathy in my feet and arms. Eventually I made the decision to travel to a world-renowned hospital with a team of specialists dedicated to treating Sjogren's patients. I made an appointment to see the only physician in the country who is board certified in rheumatology, neurology, and internal medicine. While there, I would also see an ophthalmologist and ENT specialist. I needed to wait five months for this appointment and so my local rheumatologist prescribed yet another DMARD in the mean time in hopes of it working without side effects.

Just sixteen days after starting this new drug, I began to feel sick with what I assumed was a stomach bug. Over the course of the next two days I grew sicker by the hour, but somehow never had the presence of mind to connect it with my new medication. I was scheduled to return to the rheumatologist for bloodwork four weeks after starting the medication, but was happy that this particular drug did not have a tendency to affect my liver like the previous two, allowing me to return "wine-gulping" to the "cheese-consuming-mouse-fearing-punctuation-flinging-celtic-and-Buddha-loving paradox that is me." At some point during the third day of what was now a ferocious stomach illness, a light bulb went off in my head. I realized the fact that being on an immunosuppressant may not only increase my susceptibility to becoming ill, it may prevent me from getting better as well. I then decided that it would be prudent to ask

Michael and Megan to bring me to the emergency room.

Little did I know that that was the smartest decision of my life. Little did I know that if I had made the decision *not* to go to the ER, it may well have been the *last* decision I would ever make in my life.

Once that worry about immunosuppressants came in my head, I could not let it go. I remember trying to hold it together during the interminable time it took to get to the triage room while Michael parked the car. I repeatedly instructed Megan that she needed to tell the nurses that I was on an immunosuppressant. "I am on an immunosuppressant. I am on an immunosuppressant! I AM ON AN IMMUNOSUPPRESSANT!!!" Once those words came out of my mouth in that triage room, I honestly don't remember much else. I do remember thinking that I must be verifiably ill because they rushed me down to an ER bay where a nurse and resident were waiting for me and began working on me immediately.

The next few hours and days were a fantastic blur between hallucination and reality. I had entered the hospital with septic shock – the third and final stage of a sepsis infection – and thankfully the staff in the emergency room recognized it immediately, for septic shock proves to be fatal to more than half of the patients who enter this phase. My temperature was above 103 degrees, my heart rate was very high, and my blood pressure was dangerously low. Initial blood tests revealed that most of my organs, like my kidneys and liver, had stopped functioning; sparing the little strength my body had left for my heart and brain. My lips and fingers turned blue from lack of oxygen and a blotchy rash appeared on my skin. Blood tests also revealed that my white blood count had been drastically reduced by that medicine I had been taking for just sixteen days (a very, very rare reaction to this drug) and my body had no way to fight this yet-unknown infection that was flooding through my system.

With countless bags of fluids and antibiotics flowing through IVs in each arm, and blood pressure drugs running through a central line into a vein in my neck, I eventually stabilized. Over the course of the next five days I slowly recovered, as my organs began functioning properly and the hallucinations stopped. No more John Philip Souza marches playing in my bed or imaginary stairs in my room in the "step-down" unit. I patiently accepted visitors while I was scantily clad in an institutional gown and (let's call it what it was) hospital issued diaper. Wearing a bra or pajama pants wasn't even possible, for I was monitored and wired from head to toe. At some point I had as many as seven IV bags hooked up to my pole.

Once home and still healing, I slowly began to grasp what it was that had happened to me. I heard the words "septic shock" and realized that I had dodged a huge bullet, for even though I had heard those words in the emergency room, they had held no significance to me. I was all set to die fat, dumb, and happy. I had surrendered control the second the IMMUNOSUPPRESANT word had been made known to the triage team and didn't regain it again until well after I was released.

Recovery was slow: very, very slow. Never one to have much stamina, I was now officially weak on top of it. Still, I had three months to wait for my series of appointments with the Sjogren's specialists, and this gave time for my brain and body to heal.

It also gave me time to put a new lingerie edict into effect. Although my mother taught me to make sure I wore clean underwear in case I was ever in an automobile accident, she neglected to inform me to never let my supply of acceptable panties drop below the number ten in the unlikely event I were deathly ill with a stomach bug for days before I was admitted to a hospital for a five-day stay. I can't help but think that if I had landed in that unlucky percentage of those who *didn't* survive septic shock, my friends at the funeral home would have been forced to bury me in disposable underwear supplied by the hospital. And who, I ask you, wants to be clad like that on judgment day?

Overlapping Illnesses

Shortly before my scheduled appointments, Kaitlyn, Leah and I attended the annual National Sjogren's Patient Conference which was held outside of Philadelphia. (Unfortunately Megan couldn't attend.) Beyond the thrill of meeting other Sjogren's patients and learning about different aspects of the disease from premier physicians throughout the country, I had the pleasure of introducing myself to one of the presenters – the very specialist who I was scheduled to see that following Tuesday.

I cannot tell you the difference that particular appointment has made in my life. Three skin punch biopsies were taken which verified the fact that my small-fiber neuropathy was not only present, but significant. A subsequent nerve conduction study then showed that I had acquired a mild large-fiber neuropathy – neuropathy which was not present in an identical study just six months prior. What's more, extensive blood tests came back with all sorts of unexpected abnormalities and antibodies: One was an indicator of aggressive rheumatoid arthritis (RA), others pointed to lupus, and still others to scleroderma and pernicious anemia. All of these tests had been negative when run by my local rheumatologist three years earlier. I am still undergoing further testing to rule out both scleroderma and pernicious anemia, but my new diagnosis of lupus and rheumatoid arthritis now qualifies me as having overlapping multiple autoimmune disease syndrome.

Rheumatoid Arthritis

While I am not at all pleased to have acquired two new diseases, the diagnosis of rheumatoid arthritis has some advantages when it comes to treatment. Rheumatoid arthritis is a chronic inflammation of the lining of the joints, leading to pain and swelling typically in the hands and the feet. RA is also a disease that can affect other parts of your body and produce extreme fatigue. With an estimated 1.5 million people diagnosed with RA, it is one of the most prevalent autoimmune disease and has been the focus of many research studies and interest by the pharmaceutical companies. Treatment for RA has greatly advanced in the last 30 years and the outlook has greatly improved for those, like me, with newly detected RA. These advances have made it possible to stop, or at least slow the progression of joint damage. Starting these medications as soon as possible helps prevent joints from having permanent damage.

Some of these recent advances in the treatment of RA may also be helpful in treating Sjogren's Syndrome but have not been specifically studied in Sjogren's patients and so the treatments (often extremely expensive) are not approved by insurance companies. My additional diagnosis of both RA and lupus means that I now qualify for treatment with these advanced biologic drugs. My rheumatologist/neurologist has prescribed a drug given by intravenous infusion because I have acquired a more aggressive form of RA; one that absolutely needs to be treated as soon as possible. Once again, I feel fortunate that the diagnosis came before the onset of severe symptoms and my prognosis is good. So, too, for the addition of lupus. I have not developed any specific symptoms or complications of lupus, but we now know to be on the lookout for them. Although Sjogren's and lupus are quite similar in nature (with the exception of dry eyes and mouth) I will be watched and followed more closely for complications which would not normally affect a Sjogren's patient.

So how was it that I came to acquire all of these new antibodies in my blood? Why was it that I developed large fiber neuropathy in addition to the small fiber neuropathy? It is my guess that my experience with septic shock sent my immune system into a tailspin – causing increased neuropathy and autoimmune processes. Again, it's only a guess, but it remains the most plausible theory to me.

12. Family Resemblances

Think and wonder.
Wonder and think.

– Dr. Seuss

If I have done my job correctly you must now be shaking your head and wondering, "Are these diseases hereditary? And, if so, why are they all sick with different diseases?"

The answers to these questions are not definitive, but shrouded instead in murky phrases like, "researchers believe" or "scientists think". That's because there has not been one specific gene linked to autoimmune diseases. In all probability, there are several genes that increase an individual's susceptibility to autoimmune disease.

The National Institute of Health (NIH) phrases it this way:

> No one is sure what causes autoimmune diseases. In most cases, a combination of factors is probably at work. For example, you might have a genetic tendency to develop a disease and then, under the right conditions, an outside invader like a virus might trigger it.

The American Autoimmune Related Disease Association (AARDA) states:

> The ability to develop an autoimmune disease is determined by a dominant genetic trait that is very common (20 percent of the population) that may present in families as different autoimmune diseases within the

same family. The genetic predisposition alone does not cause the development of autoimmune diseases. It seems that other factors need to be present as well in order to initiate the disease process.

However, it is not a particular autoimmune disease; it is generally a tendency to autoimmunity. One family member may have lupus, another family member may have Sjogren's disease, a third member of the family may have rheumatoid arthritis.

Sounds familiar. Does it not?

And as far as my own primary disease in concerned, the National Institute of Arthritis and Musculoskeletal and Skin Diseases reports:

Researchers think Sjogren's syndrome is caused by a combination of genetic and environmental factors. Several different genes appear to be involved, but scientists are not certain exactly which ones are linked to the disease, because different genes seem to play a role in different people. Simply having one of these genes will not cause a person to develop the disease. Some sort of trigger must activate the immune system.

Scientists think that the trigger may be a viral or bacterial infection. It might work like this: a person who has a Sjogren's-associated gene gets a viral infection. The virus stimulates the immune system to act, but the gene alters the attack, sending fighter cells (lymphocytes) to the glands of the eyes and mouth. Once there, the lymphocytes attack healthy cells, causing the inflammation that damages the glands and keeps them from working properly. This is an example of autoimmunity. These fighter cells are supposed to die after their attack in a natural process called apoptosis, but in people with Sjogren's Syndrome, they continue to attack, causing further damage. Scientists think that resistance to apoptosis may be genetic.

So simply put, researchers do not know for sure, but all evidence collected to date points to the fact that the tendency to acquire an autoimmune disease runs in families. Yet family clustering is soft data – not scientific fact.

In the case of my own cluster, I firmly believe that my family tree has developed deep roots which foster the tendency towards autoimmunity. No hard data is needed for me – the evidence gathered in my own life experience is clear and convincing. I have three daughters and two brothers who have been affected by autoimmunity. What layman would need more data than that?

Megan developed lupus after struggling with the streptococcus virus, Leah's Guillain-Barre began with her encounter with the influenza virus and bronchitis, and – although the antibodies belonging to Sjogren's Syndrome were already poised and set to go – my own battle with the flu set the disease flying into action. God himself only knows what processes my experience with septic shock sent flying in my body as well.

What's more, I fear that some of those who are not presently sick may yet encounter their particular environmental trigger. That trigger can come at any age – at twelve, twenty-two, fifty-two, or eighty-two. What would happen if my four other siblings acquire autoimmune diseases? What if my nieces and nephews have inherited my bizarre "aunt-i-bodies"?

As much as I wish it weren't true, I believe that Kaitlyn's spondyloarthritis will prove to be the precursor to a systemic autoimmune disease of her own, such as rheumatoid arthritis. In fact, you might say that all three of my daughters are still in various stages of uncertainty regarding just where their disease processes will land.

And with this bit of knowledge comes an unwanted feeling of personal guilt. I know in my heart that I could not have foreseen or prevented these illnesses, but I feel guilty nonetheless. Not only do I have to watch my daughters suffer, I have to live with the fact that their illnesses have come from me.

Because of me.

Part Two: Living with Autoimmunity

Drying My Tears

136

13. A Litany of Laments

I'm telling you this 'cause you're one of my friends.
My alphabet starts where your alphabet ends.

– Dr. Seuss

Although autoimmune diseases vary widely and, so too, their symptoms and complications, I believe that my battle with Sjogren's Syndrome could be viewed as a model of sorts for what it is like to live with an autoimmune disease. And while no one person could ever be said to be "typical," I know that others will be able to learn from my experiences with Sjogren's. Physicians, spouses, children, therapists, friends, and fellow patients can certainly benefit from hearing from those whose diseases are often overlooked or misunderstood.

So how can I begin to explain this strange and whimsically-named illness to others who cannot see anything wrong on the outside? What exactly is it like to live with a Swedish Man's Name?

To borrow a quote from Aristotle, the most startling thing I have discovered about living with Sjogren's is that, "The whole is greater than the sum of its parts." Yes, I have dry mouth and the GERD and swallowing issues which accompany it. Yes, I have dry eyes and all of the discomfort that it brings. I also experience pain, burning, and numbness from neuropathy in my hands and feet. Indeed, I have pain affecting almost every joint and muscle in my body. And for sure I have fatigue in spades. Any one of these conditions on their own would be difficult – ranging from pesky to taxing – but to experience the synergistic blend of all of these ailments every moment of every day is nothing short of life-altering.

Sjogren's is known as a disease of "flares" but I tend never to use the word when referring to the state of my disease. I honestly could not tell you if this is because I have never experienced a period of time that is bad enough to be considered a flare, or I have never felt good enough to consider myself out of one. I know that on some days some of my symptoms might be better than others, but I have yet to hit a day when the stars have magically aligned themselves and I could say that I actually feel "good." No, the feelings of pain and malaise which come with this disease which bears a Swedish man's name are such that they permeate every aspect of my life each and every day.

And it all begins with waking up.

My first sensation upon every rude awakening is a strange combination of pain and dryness. If you want to attempt to understand the parched feeling in my mouth each morning, just envision yourself as having spent the night with your dentist's gurgley-sucking thing in your open mouth all night long. Not a bit of saliva to be found. I cannot close my mouth without my lips sticking together and my tongue plastering itself to the roof of my mouth.

If you care to understand the dryness in my eyes, just imagine the sandman visiting you during the night but instead of sprinkling enchanted sand he has used sandpaper on the inside of your eyelids. And this particular dryness is something you can feel before even attempting to open your eyes. I know from painful past mistakes that I can only open my eyes with eye drops close in hand, for the abrasions on my corneas are ripped open over and over again when I raise my eyelids each morning.

As for the pain? It could be anywhere. If I have somehow slept with my fingers closed, they would be the first to declare their dismay. If not, it may be my shoulders complaining because I had the nerve to sleep upon them. (Most mornings I need to use my left arm to physically raise my right arm from the bed in order to get moving.) And speaking of nerves, the nerves in my feet are sure to let me know, here and now, that they will resist any attempt to be stuffed into shoes or socks throughout the day ahead.

Good morning world! It's time to get on with my day. But when I say "on", I often mean *on the couch. . .*

The best simile I can use to explain the malaise I feel is this: It's like the last day of a routine sickness for regular people. You wake up feeling better than you did the day before. The fever, sneezing, or vomiting are gone at long last and you say to yourself, "I'm going to get out of bed, take a proper shower, and try to vacuum some of that errant dog hair that's been accumulating in mountains since I've been sick." And so you do. After the shower, you're quite exhausted and look a little green around the gills, but you're determined to go on. Yet after a quick attempt at the minutest bit of housework you think, "Sweet Jesus! I never knew that vacuuming had been elevated to an Olympic sport!"

And at times you find yourself quickly back in bed – all the stamina you once possessed now sucked up by your battle with the vacuum and feeling like a musher who lost the *I-Did-A-Clean* to the dog hair.

Well that, my friends, is the battle that an autoimmuner fights every day. But despite the pitfalls, I have learned that I need to force myself to move on with my day – to pay bills, make sure there is food for my family, and give myself time out of my home so I don't turn into a recluse.

Others (not I, thank God) are dealing with serious and life-threatening conditions. Yet I carry around the knowledge that the other shoe could drop at any moment: that I am 30 times more likely than the average person to develop lymphoma and, because of my crazy antibodies, have a significant chance of suffering a stoke or pulmonary embolism over the course of my life. And on the opposite end of the spectrum, I have been told at times that my blood is not clotting fast enough and I'm susceptible to bleeding events. Does anyone really understand *that*?

The rest of this chapter will be dedicated to particular symptoms that I call my *Litany of Laments*. These include joint pain, muscle aches, fatigue, nerve pain, dryness, sleep disturbances, and something I like to refer to as the *Pain Train*. There is also another phrase which rhymes with "drain clog" and seems to be a common complaint among those with various autoimmune diseases. I have read about the two little words which comprise this phrase, but do not speak them out loud because I fear that if I plant a seed I might just grow a beanstalk.

Feeling Sabulous

If you look up the word "sabulous" in a dictionary, you will see that it's an authentic word meaning sandy or gritty. I believe it is the preferred way to refer to my dryness instead of the phrase "sicca symptoms." Why would I want to be reminded, yet again, that I am "sick-a?"

I would much rather feel sabulous.

Whichever the phraseology, I live with this dryness every day. As I have already indicated, I wake up each morning in a parched state which is all-but-impossible to describe. I need to be extremely vigilant in the protocol for my eye health – employing lid scrubs, warm compresses, sleeping goggles, and countless applications of eye drops throughout the day.

Crying, too, has become ancient history. I imagine that you have never thought about what a life without tears would be like; to be the only one at a funeral dispensing drops *into* your eyes instead of letting them out. Tears are cleansing and crying is cathartic. When first diagnosed, my eyes were dry but I could still call up some tears when needed. As my disease has progressed, I have lost the ability to produce emotionally-charged tears and a strong burning pain arrives when those tears would normally begin to well up in my eyes. Once the rest of my body feels this pain, it usually shuts off the crying mechanism, deciding that there can be no benefit to going ahead with the entire reaction. And if, perchance, a tear or two slides by the Sjogren's sentries? I treasure that drop well beyond the time it evaporates from my face; tracing its bittersweet track with my finger like the bereaved placing roses on a gravesite.

As for my dry mouth symptoms, a whole army of remedies is deployed to combat them – sips of water, mouth sprays, lozenges, chewing gum, and slow-release tablets. Do they work? Not particularly. Do they provide relief? For the short term. I use a saline nasal spray in my nose and a menthol-based gel for my lips. Truth be told, I also take that saline spray and use it as a mist for my face and upper chest.

There are medications which help to produce saliva and

sometimes increase tear production as well, but neither my dentist nor rheumatologist feel they would be right for me. Plugs are often used to prevent tears from draining from eyes, but – in my case – my tear ducts have already closed on their own and any attempt at plugging them is unsuccessful. There are other measures that can be taken for helping dry eye and healing corneal erosions and I am currently waiting for an appointment with a cornea specialist.

Joint and Muscle Pain

Before the onset of my own disorder, I knew that my daughters suffered joint and muscle pain. I had often witnessed all three holding their hands up against each others in a quest to find out whose joints were the most swollen. (Kaitlyn was usually the winner of this competition.) There was no need for a barometer in our house, for those girls could tell us when a rain or snow storm was on its way. And many was the morning I entered Megan's room to rouse her out of bed, only to hear her beg me to bring whichever NSAID she happened to be taking at the time because her joints were so painful she could not get out of bed.

My daughters have swum through a veritable sea of non-steroidal anti-inflammatory drugs. All have been placed on plaquenil. Kaitlyn and Leah have also tried another DMARD. Megan is now also on one of the newer biologic drugs delivered by weekly injection.

Before my diagnosis, I knew that my joints were becoming increasingly tender when I first got out of bed, that my ankles and knees were beginning to hurt when I negotiated stairs, and that genuflecting at work (the catholic curtsy) was getting harder and harder to perform each day.

Sometime after my diagnosis I discovered the word "pain", but I certainly didn't want to apply it to my situation. I could easily use the phrase "joint pain" when speaking of my condition, but I never wanted to say that I was "in" pain. Something just seemed wrong about that. I know of so many others whose medical challenges are more difficult than mine. Their diseases are life threatening, while mine is simply life changing.

Here's a little secret: I may not want to use the word, but I live it.

I experience some sort of pain from the moment I wake up in the morning until I wake up twenty-four hours later. Pain weaves and glides its way though my body throughout the night: when I roll over in bed and feel my shoulders, hips, and knees hurting, when I hobble to the bathroom on throbbing ankles, and when my fingers and toes begin to pound. Did you know that pain is a nocturnal creature? I have never known it to sleep.

This pain goes right to the bone. It makes me think twice about getting up out of a chair, doing laundry, climbing the stairs to the bedroom, holding onto a steering wheel, or typing on my laptop.

Nerve Pain

I admit that it is sometimes hard for me to differentiate between joint, muscle, and nerve pain. The three are often combined in my case. When I have been on a prednisone regime, the joint and muscle pain due to inflammation inherent with Sjogren's practically disappears, leaving me with what I assume is then nerve pain. And I have learned that all nerve pain is not equal. It sears. It burns. It zaps. It aches. It crawls. It pings. It is both ice cold and blazing hot, predictable and haphazard. As you read about *The Pain Train* later in this chapter, you will be treated to some samplings of the intermittent nerve pain I experience, but for now I will concentrate on the predicable pain from small fiber neuropathy.

I assume that the two medications I take to address this pain have alleviated the hurtful process somewhat, yet I still wake up each night with pain in my feet and legs; much like the sensation that they have been burned. I often stare at the tops of those feet in disbelief that these innocent-looking appendages – freezing to the touch during daylight hours – are not covered in third-degree burns; for that is exactly how they feel.

The personal remedies I have developed for dealing with my nocturnal pain would make a casual observer laugh. I have given up all hope of ever sleeping with a top sheet tucked in and have moved my bed so that, when needed, I can twist, turn, and maneuver myself into such a shape that either the tops or bottoms of my feet and fingers can rest lightly up against the cool bedroom wall. Were you under the mistaken impression that I was still sharing a bed with my husband of 30 years? No, my midnight dryness, snoring, restless pain, and Goldilocks-like search for just the right bed have landed me permanently in the Zen room.

I would venture to guess that, spouse or not, you have never played footsie with your bedroom wall in the middle of the night. Nor have you ever, in your wildest dreams, thought that that very same wall could serve as a painkiller. What's more, I have to admit that I have lately developed a sort of amorous affection for the cold tiles of the bathroom floor for they, too, have also become a welcome analgesic on many an agonizing night. I invite you to try it sometime to catch the sensation. If I, with my limited ability to sense temperature, have found it helpful, I can only imagine how good it would feel for you.

Lately I have come to another discovery. I often wake up throughout the night or first thing in the morning with a type of discomfort which I can only describe as residing under every inch of my skin. It is a tingling receptor-like pain which I described in an earlier chapter as being like a "skin ache," but now I am going to change my own description of this discomfort to "feeling like I am going to spontaneously combust." Heretofore I assumed this combustion pain was the result of those little fighter cells working overtime while I slumbered, yet now I know that it, too, is a type of nerve pain associated with small fiber neuropathy.

The Pain Train

This particular term is a phenomenon that may be a tad bit difficult for an outsider to grasp, but I beg you to accept my explanation. Forget all about *The Polar Express* and *The Little Engine that Could*, *The Pain Train* is real! It is a unique occurrence which is characterized by its very randomness. The train pulls into my station early in the morning every few days. Believe me when I tell you that this is not a train one would ever hop on voluntarily.

How to explain?

I imagine *The Pain Train* like this: A renegade hobo has jumped, uninvited, on an invisible train inside my body and decides to take a joy ride, meandering at will, and wreaking havoc at every stop along the way. I haven't quite determined whether this havoc is of a neurological, gastroenterological, or vascular nature – most likely a combination of all three – but this invader is determined to create mayhem wherever he travels.

Here is just a small sampling of one of his haphazard itineraries:

Mr. Hobo jumps on board and decides to stop in my gallbladder which he mistakenly views as a bowling alley, deciding to knock back a few games with my hibernating gallstones. The pain comes in waves as those newly-awakened stones land strike after strike, sparing me no pain. I, however, recognize these twinges for what they are. I should have had my gallbladder removed years ago.

After a while, he gets bored, jumping back on the gastroenterological track, landing right in the weak spot of my diverticula pockets where he quickly morphs into a construction worker with a jackhammer, causing minutes or hours of sharp, unrelenting pain.

I sometimes thank my lucky stars that our friend has been diagnosed with attention deficit disorder because he soon switches train lines altogether and travels to my lungs, causing pain with each breath for about five minutes or so – just long enough to leave me worried that a blood clot has traveled to my lungs.

Very shortly, I start to develop pain in my left shoulder and – even if my rheumatologist has given me a cortisone shot to ward off the throbbing which hangs around even when my shoulder is not in use – Hoboman decides to leave some of his minions there to stand up and scream whenever my arm reaches a certain height.

The renegade freeloader may then take a detour back to my large intestine to create more mayhem or opt to travel instead to the hinterlands of my salivary glands in order to practice his boxing skills.

As you might imagine, Hoboman has the most difficulties as he approaches the terminal parts of my body. As he travels down the inside of my left leg – in what I'm convinced is the neuropathic subway of my system – he produces a significant amount of searing pain along the way.

Once he reaches my ankle he has a critical choice to make: Should he proceed at once through the tarsal tunnel? Or is the general traffic less congested on the outlying path? Being from the greater New York area, Mr. Hobo instinctively knows that the tunnel route is rarely the better choice – in this case due to the backup of peripheral neuropathy – so he chooses to attack my feet via the sural nerve and lands squarely and definitively in my left pinkie toe. Ouch! I'm talking a searing and pounding sensation for a good five minutes or so as he discovers the fun run has literally reached its end and attempts to reroute his itinerary back to the more densely populated areas of my body.

Yet sometimes he detours and ends in the terminal of my big toe. At other times, he lands in the knuckles of my toes – playing all five of them like a set of steel drums.

Similarly, if that rebel decides to travel down my arm, he often chooses my left arm, deciding to shoot down it repetitively; an Olympic competitor on a bob-sled run. Once he reaches the carpal tunnel, he once-again opts for the singular route of the ulnar nerve and lands squarely in my left pinkie finger. The pain pulses throughout my hand causing me to shake it repeatedly.

Lately I have become convinced that this man has become licensed as an official flamethrower, as he stands at the top of my right leg and pitches his burning torch right at the top of my right foot. This pain is so intense that I am unable to maintain my composure while he lobs eight or ten of these weapons at me.

Now back to a knee. . . or a hip. . . or ear . . . wherever it is that our Hobo has decided to travel next.

I have no weapons with which to fight him and can only wait out his visits – hoping against hope that he will find a great need to sleep off his joy ride or hop onto someone else's train for a few days.

Sleep Disturbances

There is absolutely no way of describing my sleeping patterns to you, except to say that they don't exist.

On an average night I get about 11 hours of sleep, but that would be a night when insomnia hasn't hit and left me awake for a period of two or three hours. It would also mean a night when I'm not suffering from depletion and fatigue, in which case a comatose state of slumber would then unfold for 15 continuous hours despite my family's best efforts to shake me out of bed.

I recently had an at-home sleep study done which revealed that, although I thought I had experienced a full night's sleep, I had a calculated sleep efficiency rating of 65, which means that I was only truly asleep 65 percent of the time I was in sleep mode. The rest of the time was spent on the very top surface encountering awakening and arousals. While an average sleeper would have entered REM five or six times during the night, I only entered it twice. On one of these occasions I immediately woke up, leaving me with only one real REM session.

The sleep study also revealed the truth of what my husband has been telling me for years and verifies the reason I toss and turn in the Zen room instead of sharing a bed with him. I snored 60 percent of the time I was asleep, and 13 percent was classified as loud snoring.

Readers who want to remain my friend will never mention these results to him.

Although I end up with erratic types of sleep, my bedtime preparation is always consistent. First, I fill and start my humidifier to ensure I am surrounded by moist air. I stage a multitude of pillows in just the right places in and around my twin-sized bed. I spray saline spray in my nostrils, swab the inside of my freshly-brushed mouth with a PH-balanced gel, and spread a menthol balm on my lips. I then don my wrist splints and drop thick eye drops in my eyes before covering them with rubber sleep goggles lest any air sneak into my eyes through a tiniest slit in a closed lid.

Sounds like I'm readying myself for some fisticuffs with the sandman instead of settling in for a cozy night's sleep in my Zen room, now doesn't it?

We have just uncovered the very dichotomy which runs through my life. I bathe my bed in fluffy white comforters to make it look inviting, but cannot use a top sheet unless I care to be sporting it as a toga by morning. I spray an aromatherapy mist on my bedclothes, but still pull on wrist splints as I would boxing gloves. I stage no less than six pillows in various areas of my tiny twin bed, only to end up using them as punching bags in my battle with insomnia. All sorts of preventive measures are employed to pretend I will be slumbering in a rain forest, only to wake up somewhere in the Sahara Desert around 3:00 a.m. with my mouth parched, lids glued to my eyes, and thousands of ants crawling under my skin.

I have already regaled you with my wall-hugging antics and will not do so again, but I would like to tell you a bit about my sleep poses. The practice of yoga includes a series of poses whose names often represent the look of the individual while holding the pose – like the *Lotus Pose*. Tai chi also has exquisitely-named movements whose very unfolding is meant to replicate that found in nature, like my personal favorite, *White Crane Spreads Its Wings*. Akin to these two eastern practices, my personal slumber poses also represent my bodily shape while attempting to sleep.

Even though I go to bed with splints to keep my wrists immobilized, I can't help but think that I would benefit greatly from an old fashioned straight jacket, for as much as I love the sound of the word "akimbo", I cannot sleep that way unless –

thanks to my carpal tunnel neuropathy – I want to wake up countless times throughout the night with arms and hands sound asleep.

Hence my personal sleep poses.

The pose I most often employ is *Teacher, Call on Me* as I lie on my left side and extend my entire left arm above my head. My right arm then remains resting on the side of my body. Once I grow tired of this, I roll into the *Put Your Hands Up* pose with both arms raised over my head, or attempt *Attention Soldier* with arms glued to my side. Knowing that neither of these poses are ideal for one who others deem a snorer, I then roll over into my *Miniature Golf* pose, or undertake *Embrace Pillows* instead.

The next time I have a sleepless night I plan to work a little harder on my pose nomenclature, finding beautiful items in nature to replace the very mundaneness of my pose designations. Keep in mind that my feet are very often plastered to the wall, so I have all sorts of options open to me like, *One Armed Mermaid Glides Noiselessly though Cool Waters*.

If you thought you were finished being treated to my nocturnal disturbances, you were wrong.

Did you ever have a dream that you had to go to the bathroom and wake up to discover that the urge was real? I now have the added benefit of different real-time physical discomforts invading my dreams and turning them into nightmares, like the one that opened this very book. I dream about finding my mouth stuck together so that I cannot speak or scream, or about chewing shards of glass and mirrors. I then abruptly wake up with my mouth so parched that I grab my mouth spray immediately. I dream about not being able to breathe and wake up with my chest aching. I dream about armies of ant bites and swarms of bee stings and wake up with pain under my skin. I dream all sorts of nightmarish scenarios only to be woken by my husband who has heard my terrifying screams from his own bedroom across the hall.

When my children were little and would wake with a nightmare I would place my forehead against theirs for several seconds, promising them I was taking all of those bad images away – transferring them to my own brain which they erroneously believed capable of handling their bad thoughts. The first few times Michael woke me from a night terror I longed for him to do the same for me, feeling strangely bereft as he left my room in a perfunctory sleep-haze to return to his own.

Yet I know that – no matter how big or strong – no one is able to carry these thoughts, feelings, or sensations away for me. They are mine to keep.

Fatigue

While I know it is quite impossible for me to explain the overwhelming sensation of fatigue to someone who hasn't experienced it firsthand, I will attempt nonetheless.

Fatigue, simply put, is the crushing feeling which washes over you and makes you feel as if you simply cannot spend two more minutes of your life in an upright position.

Have you ever been in church and found yourself gazing longingly at your pew; madly fighting the urge to succumb to its sirens' song inviting you to lie down and sleep? Or attended a meeting and fantasized about ways to stretch your body out upon the row of chairs lining the edge of the room? If you have, I welcome you to my club. If you haven't, you may be thinking, "What's the big deal? I've been tired before. How can I not understand?"

Yes, I also knew what it was like to be tired, to work a 14 hour day, be in charge of a large event, or suffer from a string of sleepless nights. I just never knew what it would feel like to begin each and every day of my life feeling like I had just completed all of the above. I lived a full 54 years on this planet without feeling the "tiredness-beyond-tired" type of depletion I now experience.

In truth, I still feel tired sometimes. The rest of the time I feel fatigued.

While many autoimmune diseases often bring with them a sense of fatigue, Sjogren's appears to be one of the worst offenders. Fatigue can be difficult for scientists to both define and measure. A recent study published in the American College of Rheumatology journal using the widely accepted FACIT questionnaire, found that roughly 30 percent of primary Sjogren's patients had severe fatigue. Of those who suffered from fatigue, there was a stronger correlation to those who also had depression, arthritis, impaired sleep quality, and a personality trait characterized by an inability to deal with stress. (Sound like anyone we know?) But while scientists may be getting better at studying fatigue, they still have absolutely nothing with which to fight it.

I have always been a sleeper, requiring a good nine hours of sleep each night. I also was a first-rate napper, able to fly off to the land of nod on a whim. But the exhaustion to which I now surrender demands sleep from me like a robber at gunpoint. And the naps which I now take are no longer of a carefree flowing nature, but those of a drowning victim fighting to resurface. Taking a nap every day may sound quite luxurious and I dare say a bit decadent. Those who do not know better may find themselves envying my free time and limited responsibilities. Yet as any toddler will tell you, a nap is only fun if it has not been forced upon you.

It is not just one type of exhaustion or weariness I'm speaking of here. This sensation can be multi-faceted and hit with different intensity at different times. I invite you to join me on a walk down fatigue lane:

> **The Oh No, I'm Awake! Tiredness** – This is the one I face each and every morning. Sleep? Did I really sleep? I know I spent time in my bed, because I distinctly remember waking up about 25 times throughout the night but the word "rested" somehow just doesn't seem to apply.
>
> **The Bone Tired Fatigue** – This is the one that comes from dealing with joint and muscle pain. All of that *ouch-ing* drains my energy and makes getting from here to there a feat of great proportions.
>
> **The Lead Foot Weariness** – Having a lead foot usually refers to one who has the propensity to drive fast, but there is nothing fast about this. It feels like something or someone, is literally weighing me down – forcing me to move in slow motion.
>
> **The All-But-Surgically-Attached-to-My-Bed Sleepiness** – These are the days when I just can't wake up; when my children or husband try to rouse me from my bed. I respond and tell them I'll be up shortly, and drop back into a *d-e-e-p* sleep within seconds; unable to move from the

bed.

The I Emptied Half of the Dishwasher and Need to Rest Exhaustion (a.k.a. **I Just Took a Shower Fatigue**) – All of that up-and-down with my arms, spine, and head. Exhausting. This particular fatigue is somewhat akin to the **I Vacuumed the Living Room Depletion** – sucks the life right out of me.

The In Your Face Fatigue – This is the one that brings cobwebs to your brain, glassiness to your eyes, and a sense that you are already asleep to your very face. I have no choice but to surrender to this one – for where the head goes, the body must follow.

And then my friends, there is the BIG one:

The Walking Dead Wipeout – This is the one that descends in a heartbeat and drops me to my knees. This fatigue begins by turning my leg muscles to rubber, spreads by squeezing the life-sustaining air out of my lungs, and completes the wipeout by leaving me with a blank facial affect and a brain which can only think of three little words in one specific order:

Must.

Lie.

Down.

Here's a short story to demonstrate my point:

Because of the unpredictability in our family planning, Leah's birthday lands just four days after Christmas – a fact that seems to surprise me every year. Her due date was January 19th after all, and let me simply state for the record that it would be extremely helpful to the woman who suffered through those unproductive labor pains if all involved would agree to celebrate her lifeday on her due date instead of her arrival date. But because no one agrees with me, her birthday last year arrived four days after the Christmas hoopla and was no different than previous ones.

Thanks to online purchasing and a please-note-dear-daughters-that-you-are-only-getting-one-gift-so-you-better-make-it-a-big-one rule, I had breezed through the horrors of Christmas shopping with a few clicks of my mouse.

But because birthdays are birthdays and single-focused mothers are aptly named, I suddenly found that I needed to procure a lifeday gift for my daughter. Leah, thankfully, knew just what she wanted so on the big day itself, I gathered up my credit card and traveled to exactly one department in one major store in the one mall close to us and found her one present. Keep in mind, the Christmas return season was in full swing so I had to wait in line for about ten minutes before I got to the register.

I had entered that store directly from the parking lot and didn't intend to see the inside of that mall again until the lifeday girl turned fifty, but it suddenly dawned on me that I needed to purchase a card and wrapping paper. (Who was I kidding? By this time I knew I was destined to shove the gift into a gift bag, but I knew from previous attempts that my precious daughter did not like sharing her birthday with the Christ Child and that any attempt of disguising a birthday gift in leftover Christmas trimmings would be shunned.) I was beginning to feel myself dragging – somewhat akin to the **Lead Foot Fatigue** noted above – but nevertheless I trudged down the corridor of the mall and into the card store. There are never many return shoppers in a card store, so my time there was short and sweet. Yet as I was standing at the register waiting to pay, the infamous death knell rang, my eyes glazed over, and I was officially hit with the **Walking Dead Wipeout.**

All that remained was to simply make my way back through the mall and out the door to my car.

Try telling my limbs and lungs that.

I still thank my lucky stars for those swanky leather chairs that they now put in malls. I grabbed the first one I saw and tried to calculate how many steps were left from there to my car. When I realized that those steps were more than I could count on two hands, I tried my best to flag down the stop-in-the-name-of-the-mall officer for a piggy-back ride on his motor scooter, but he buzzed past me too quickly to see my distress.

What to do?

Next, I sent a text to my husband informing him I was being held against my will in a leather chair at the mall – hoping against hope that he would come and save me, but it turns out that husbands, like mall police, are not always available for rescue missions. My husband was in a meeting and not by his phone.

The only thing I could do was to sit and rest. So that's exactly what I did. In every leather chair I saw. Even if it was thirty feet away from the one I just got out of. "Baby steps," I thought. "Teeny, tiny, baby steps."

That, my friends, is the very reason I live in fear of setting foot in a mall again, the motive for ordering all of my clothing and shoes online, and the rationale for ordering most of my groceries for home delivery. And when I do go to the local market to buy produce, fish, and – let's admit it – prepared foods, I never carry a hand cart and oh-so-politely ask the bagger or check-out clerk to reach into the abysses of that cart to pack it all up again.

If I did not, I would be sure to encounter the **I Just Emptied the Dishwasher Fatigue** in the parking lot of the store.

Drain Clog

I will use the two little words here which I have very rarely spoken aloud: the ones which rhyme with "drain clog".

Brain Fog.

This is a phrase in whose existence I heretofore refused to believe. Yet, as I typed that last sentence I misspelled *beleive*.

This is my *delemna* (correction, dilemma). I have always fancied myself a writer and – what's more – a loquacious vocabularian as well. But lately something has been wrong with my brain. I have not wanted to admit, nor even acknowledge, my newly-acquired deficits but I have somehow misplaced a good portion of my spelling ability and word-producing skills. Please note that I did not refer to it as word finding skills – I never had to find words before. They always rolled off the tips of my fingers.

If I own up to the fact that I have experienced that strange *phenomemon* (*phenomonom*) (no, *phenominom*) (let's try again, *phenonimun*) I am afraid that I will start to let down my guard and attribute all-things-goofy to this phrase. I'm afraid it will become a crutch, a mask, a shield to hide behind. A self-fulfilling *prophecty*. Those two little words will become an excuse when I forget the names of acquaintances. I will stop pretending that I remember who I told which story to. When Michael says, "You've told me that already," I will be forced to believe him for the first time in our marital existence.

People may begin to notice my difficulties and start filling in the words for me. Do you know how they always claim that your soul mate can finish your sentences for you? Please no! I've had people do that for me and it's nothing short of humiliating.

I have fought this drain clog tooth and nail. I have blamed my *percieved* shortcomings on my emotional state, my medication, my laptop, and the fact that I am no longer working. My world has grown so much smaller; why not my brain? I have even had two MRIs of my brain and an MRA of my head to ensure that there was no physical reason for this problem.

It was the process of writing this book which started to convince me of the validity of those two words. I have often waited patiently, but now admittedly with growing frustration, to try to bring a familiar word to mind. Countless times I have had to resort to the "*sylable*" – no, the "*synanym*" – no the "synonym" tool to refresh my memory. If it were not for squiggly red lines, this book would be a jumble of misspelled words. In the past two days, just knowing this chapter was in the making, I compiled a list of words which I have had trouble bringing to mind: endocrinologist, gazebo, shish kabob, cathartic, significant, irresponsible, melanoma, pragmatic, cruise control, painting, phrases, *compolication*, acquired, and disorder. I'm sure there will be many more before the book is completed.

As hard as I try to hide these shortcomings, I sometimes get caught. Earlier today I was forced to show Leah a piece of Velcro and ask her what it was called. Once I had entered the web of embarrassment, I then asked her how to spell it.

One night I came home from a dinner out with friends, mortified by my lack of conversational skills. It seemed to me that we had spent half the meal in silence, waiting as I shook my brain, or made imitative gestures, in hopes of bringing a particular word to light.

On another evening out with the same friends, we left the restaurant only to discover that it had begun to rain. We rushed to our respective cars and departed for home – all, that is, except for me. Once in my car, I could not remember how to turn the windshield wipers on. And this car, which I had owned for 18 months, was not coughing up its secrets easily. My frantic fumbling found me switching on and off rear wipers and headlights, but could not recall the magic movement which would induce those two precious wands to begin their timely tango across my front windshield. Panic descended. What to do? I decided to take a deep breath, turn the car off, and start from scratch again. Sure enough, my muscle memory proved greater than my brain recall and the rainwater quickly began its descent from my windshield, unaware of all the turmoil it had caused me.

One day the vision specialist Megan works for watched carefully as I tried to take notes on the instructions he was giving me. When I tried to write the word for the prescription eye drops I use, the pen hovered in my hand over the paper for an inordinate length of time as I attempted to write the quite-familiar word which started with an "R" – not even knowing how to begin. As I mumbled some nonsense to him about my fingers no longer writing correctly, he saw through my charade and offered to do cognitive testing and therapy on me; the same techniques he uses for concussion patients. My brilliant-Princeton-graduate-of-a-father lived the last year of his life in a nursing home due to the progression of

Alzheimer's disease; a disease which researchers now believe may have a strong connection with inflammation. I'm terrified, and know that I would benefit from baseline testing and memory and focus exercises.

If you have read this far, I sincerely hope you have picked up the fact that I am a quick-witted, competent, and sagacious woman. I am dismayed to find that something which I previously thought was nothing more than a fabrication or excuse may have been true after all. Not only true, but creeping into my life like an unwanted parasite. If I feel this way, I can't imagine what it will be like if I ever try to throw that phrase out there to explain my behavior to others.

Talk about an invisible illness!

14. Complications in Common

You're in pretty good shape for the shape you are in.

– Dr. Seuss

Once again, because our diseases are related, our family resemblances continue through some other conditions that often accompany these illnesses. You will get to hear all about them now.

Raynaud's Phenomenon

Raynaud's Phenomenon occurs when the body's blood vessels narrow more than usual in response to cold temperatures. During an attack, a person's fingers and toes change colors and go from white, to blue, to red. They usually feel cold and numb from lack of blood flow. As the attack ends and blood flow returns, fingers and toes will begin to throb and tingle and normal blood flow will return in about 15 minutes. Raynaud's Phenomenon can exist as an isolated problem or in association with any of the connective tissue disorders. It is very often found in those who suffer from lupus and Sjogren's.

If you recall, back in an earlier chapter I recounted the story about how a Raynaud's attack had the attendants in the college infirmary insisting that Kaitlyn visit the emergency room. I can only suppose that they had never seen, nor heard, of such a crazy condition.

In the big picture, the presence of Raynaud's does not affect the quality of my life in a significant way and usually just means that my feet turn cold and purple at some point each afternoon, yet I am not the only one in the family who suffers from this "phenomenon" and it seems to be worse for my daughters. Keeping hands and feet warm is usually the best defense against Raynaud's, but – as you might guess – those girls would much rather be sporting a brand new spring mani-pedi than be bundled in boots and gloves until Flag Day.

Antiphospholipid Antibody Syndrome

Antiphospholipid antibodies are present in Megan's blood as well as in my own. These antibodies often, but not always, are associated with lupus. Because these antibodies consistently appear at high levels in her blood, Megan can be labeled as having Antiphospholipid Antibody Syndrome.

These are also the antibodies which – while not tested at the time – wreaked havoc with my pregnancies; for the syndrome provokes pregnancy-related complications such as miscarriage, stillbirth, preterm delivery, and pre-eclampsia. And they are, most likely, the same antibodies which allowed that New York obstetrician to reassure my mother that she was presenting with a false-positive test for an unthinkable disease in 1951.

The correlation between lupus and false-positive results on syphilis tests was discovered in the 1940's when doctors realized that one in five lupus patients tested positive, and hence, the first, fledgling test for antiphospholipid antibodies was recognized.

Further research which identified both clotting issues and pregnancy losses did not appear again until the 1980's – just in time for these results to trickle down to the average obstetrician as I was in the midst of my own childbearing years. Although reliable blood tests were not yet in use, my own doctor felt confident enough to place me on low-dose aspirin throughout my third pregnancy.

Antiphospholipid antibodies interfere with the way an individual's blood clots in ways that are unpredictable and not completely understood (at least not by me). As any hematologist will tell you, the clotting process is a complicated tightrope walk. If your body is not able to form a blood clot quickly enough, you run the serious risk of losing too much blood. Conversely, if your blood clots too quickly or easily you run a high risk of developing deep vein thrombosis, pulmonary embolisms, or stroke. The presence of antiphospholipid antibodies in your blood makes an individual vulnerable to both types of clotting problems and it is virtually impossible to predict which clotting difficulty may develop.

Some physicians choose to do nothing when the presence of these antibodies is discovered; fearing that placing a patient on blood thinners without evidence of blood clots may contribute to a bleeding event. Others will place their patients on low dose aspirin. As I write this, I know from Megan's last visit to her rheumatologist that her antibody levels have become significantly elevated. Does this mean that she will suffer a stroke or pulmonary embolism tomorrow? It is highly unlikely, but within the realm of possibility. When young people like Megan develop thrombotic issues, the majority of them are found to have antiphospholipid antibodies at significant levels in their blood.

I try not to think of what the presence of these antibodies may signify for any potential pregnancy in Megan's future. I know that she will be placed in the high risk category and given blood thinners throughout. I hope that she will be able to enjoy her childbearing years without fear and heartache.

In many ways, I am thankful that knowledge of these antibodies was still somewhat sketchy throughout my own years of childbearing, but yet it has been a great relief to me to finally dispel the misconception which had gnawed at me throughout the first years of motherhood. My body had not been reacting to, or viewing, the presence of a fetus as a foreign invader; this was, instead, an autoimmune response like any of those we have learned about. I wasn't an "unnatural" mother who rejected my husband's very DNA inside of my womb, I was – instead – a woman who had an issue with clotting and did not know it.

I would be lying if I told you that the presence of these same antibodies in my blood doesn't cause me to worry about my own health. The thought of a blood clot, pulmonary embolism, or stroke strikes fear into my already anxiety-ridden heart. As much as I try not to worry about such things, I tend to become slightly terrified whenever *The Pain Train* causes twinges or pain in my legs or lungs.

Photosensitivity

Ultraviolet radiation emitted from the sun and some fluorescent lights can alter immune function and lead to an autoimmune response in the body and in the skin. Skin rashes and disease flares often result from exposure to the sun. Although it is true that some medications can cause skin to burn more easily, this is a reaction separate and apart from that. In Sjogren's this sun sensitivity is usually associated with the autoantibody SS-A. If you recall, the SS-A autoantibody is the very one which is positive in me.

You have heard the story about how Megan's rheumatologist emphatically insisted that she not spend time in the sun. If you recall, I lost that battle during Megan's teenage years when she decided to skip off to the beach despite my warnings. What's more, once she went off to college I'm convinced that Megan spent more time sporting those little goggles inside a tanning booth than she did donning glasses in the library. Yet somehow she never seemed to suffer any repercussions from her exposure to UV light.

That has changed in the last few years. Exposure to the sun now causes a pronounced rash to appear across her chest, yet the rash is temporary in nature; receding within an hour out of the sun. Megan also has reactive skin. An errant tag on a shirt or sweater will cause her to develop a big welt; a heating pad will leave a huge red blotch wherever it has touched her skin; exhaustion will bring a butterfly blush across her face.

My story is similar.

I used to love to soak up the sun. In my previous life, a day at the pool or beach would make me feel healthy, happy, inexplicably content. I remember returning home feeling nothing short of refreshed after spending long afternoons at the town pool or on the beach.

Almost at the same time I started experiencing my first symptoms of dryness, I noticed something strange. Whenever my arms were exposed to the sun they immediately turned bright red. This redness would subside within a half-hour of coming back inside, but it was disconcerting. During my leave of absence, the early days of May had me longing for afternoons spent on my back deck, but I quickly realized that exposure to the sun was causing me to develop a rash on my chest and upper arms.

So now I stay out of the sun altogether – wearing long sleeved clothing and a hat throughout the summer. Although I had already lost my desire to spend long days on the beach while at the family beach house, I find myself shut up inside while others enjoy their time in the sun. And if, by chance, I spend any time at a pool in a long-sleeved bathing suit, hat, and covered in sunscreen, I no longer feel refreshed or content. Instead, I am hit with **the Walking Dead Wipeout**.

Tummy Troubles

I have read that the body's entire gastrointestinal tract is approximately 30 feet long. I am quite convinced that there isn't an inch in there which hasn't caused a problem for some member of my family.

Most of us are dismayed when we enter our fifties and find it's time to subject ourselves to the ultimate in humiliation – the dreaded colonoscopy. We joke about it. We laugh. We even find humor in the fact that once we find ourselves talking about it (and who can refrain?) it means that we have become as old as our parents once were. I challenge you to find another family where two daughters have had to endure the embarrassment of undergoing colonoscopies before the age of 25.

My GERD, Barrett's esophagus, gastritis, and duodenitis are all caused by inflammation brought on by lack of saliva and other gastric juices. My diverticulitis may just have been random in nature, but whenever I hear the word "inflammation" I begin to wonder. I also have antibodies towards that intrinsic factor produced in your stomach which allows vitamin B12 to be absorbed and leads to pernicious anemia – one of the autoimmune diseases Leah suffers from.

Kaitlyn was diagnosed with a stomach ulcer at the age of 24; an ulcer most likely caused by years of use of the daily NSAIDs she takes to help alleviate the joint and muscle pain from her arthritis. As I indicated in an earlier chapter, sometimes spondyloarthropathies predate other diseases, such as psoriatic arthritis and inflammatory bowel disease. I think it would be fair to say that all three of my daughters now suffer from Irritable Bowel Syndrome but as for now, it is not yet proven that autoimmunity is responsible for their symptoms.

Hair Loss

For years I have cringed each time I peek into my daughters' shower, not only because there are 25 half-used bottles of girlie scrubs, rubs, and dubs spread throughout, but because I am inevitably treated to a display of "hair art" on the shower wall. The hair, which serves as the medium for each masterpiece, is that which has fallen out of Kaitlyn and Megan's scalps as they wash their hair.

Kaitlyn has not lived at home for many a year so I cannot tell you if she still uses the shower wall as a canvas for her paintings, but I have had the pleasure of being the sole curator of the gallery which houses Megan's works of art since she first became sick at the age of 11. Megan's once-thick head of hair has been greatly reduced since that time. I'm sure if she were to attempt to put her hair into her once-cherished pigtails, there would be less in each one than the bristles on a paintbrush.

My hairdresser tells me that the average person loses 50 strands of hair each day. As we know, my offspring could never be called average. I do not want to give you the impression that they look like those undergoing chemotherapy treatment, and – unlike those pigtail days – there are no bald spots shining through, but I am amazed that they can each lose the amount of hair they do without it becoming more noticeable.

Leah, on the other hand, has been diagnosed with a condition called alopecia areata; a common autoimmune skin disease which has caused coin-sized patches of hair loss on her scalp. With topical steroid treatment, her hair has been able to regrow, but the condition will always be with her and may reappear at some point in her life.

During the time when I was taking one particular immunosuppressant drug, my own hairbrush quickly became Enemy Number One as I experienced accelerated hair loss myself. Imagine my horror when I re-entered my bathroom after showering one day to find the first of my own splotchy and random, blotchy and tandem, designs plastered to my shower wall. I got rid of that mess quicker than a thief at a museum heist.

I am determined that there will be no reminders of all I have lost carelessly left on display for others to see.

15. The Emotional Toll

Be who you are;
say what you feel;
because those who mind don't matter,
and those who matter don't mind.

– Dr. Seuss

As I write this chapter I have been cautiously carrying my personal cup of afflictions for two years, hoping that none might spill over. I am not sure if I have something new to say that has not come to light in previous chapters, but will try my best to see what pours out.

Wheel of Misfortune

One of the things I have learned since becoming sick is just how many painful feelings I keep below the surface, waiting to percolate to the top. When, perchance, I do let down my guard and emotions spill forward, the results have often been a disaster. And a breakdown without the benefit of tears can prove to be quite comical.

I believe I started this process with what I thought was acceptance, but I now realize that I did not grasp the full meaning of what it was I was accepting. I assumed my illness would be easy because it seemed simple. "Oh this?" I thought, "I can live with this! I can hobble, cough, and nap with the best of them!"

It was new. It was novel. It was unfamiliar. I was mistaken. My illness was insidious and I was nothing short of naive.

How was I to know what I was in for? How could I foresee that I would continue to feel a little worse each day? That new symptoms would continue to appear? That the hobbling, coughing, and napping would get to be draining? The whole scene has grown very old in just two years. Perhaps my biggest fear is that this process has not reached bottom and I have no way to be certain that I can, in fact, live with this. Am I really destined to wake up each and every morning feeling like this? Will I never again feel refreshed? Renewed? Free from pain?

I would be lying if I told you that I am not sometimes envious of those families who have not been touched by misfortune. Can you imagine how I feel when I watch others living their lives to the fullest; rejoicing in happy moments and "normal" family happenings? Try as I might, I can't help but feel some sort of jealousy towards them. I know I have a supportive husband and three wonderful daughters, but sometimes I find myself wondering, "Why did these diseases descend upon my family and not theirs?"

And watching perfectly lovely and capable friends performing my former job duties with dignity and perceived ease? Resentment or envy would never be the words to describe the emotions that I feel. I can only say that it brings with it a certain sort of sadness; for they have what I no longer possess – strength, energy, and stamina.

The woman I used to be could move mountains. The woman I

have become cannot move her shopping cart through the grocery store.

I will admit right now that I am sometimes angry with others for not being attentive enough towards my plight. The Sjogren's Syndrome Foundation website has pointers on how to deal with the effects of various symptoms. The author of the page on neuropathy informs her readers that she cajoles her husband into massaging her feet each night. The last time I let my husband anywhere near one of my feet was when he had to remove my shoe to let the garter pass it at our wedding. Does anyone seriously think that I would ask him to massage my deformed feet? I would have to pay someone to do that. It's called a pedicure. And, what's more, the massage hurts. Keep your hot stones to yourself. I prefer my cold wall.

Identity Theft

"What's in a name?" you might ask.

You never know until you lose yours.

I used to be Liz Wilkey and those two little words meant a lot. Liz Wilkey was a person who did things. Countless people would need to speak with Liz, for she ran your events, booked your meetings, arranged your baptisms, and helped you through your loved ones' funerals.

Liz Wilkey was even affectionately dubbed "Know It All" by some.

Believe it or not, Liz had her peeps. Through no fault of their own, other people started to become known as "Liz Wilkey's Husband" or "Liz Wilkey's Mother."

Liz had a phone and numerous people had her number; leaving that thing buzzing, beeping, and chiming all day long. Poor Liz could barely keep that thing charged, for it seemed that her phone, like Liz, worked a good 50 hours a week.

I have had to face the fact that I am no longer that Liz Wilkey.

In truth, I no longer even have to utter those two words together at one time. I have no reason to answer a phone by reciting my name. I rarely need to call or text anyone who does not have me as a contact. When I write my name on the little sheet at a doctor's office, I am forced to write "Elizabeth". The same is true when I go to the pharmacy to pick up my prescriptions. (Who am I kidding here? Those pharmacists see me coming and start loading up a shopping cart with my family's medications. There is no anonymity in a drug store when you are their most valuable customer.)

And my phone? My phone, too, has become a silent sufferer, as entire days go by and no one attempts to contact me. I can, however, be assured of receiving one text around 7:00 p.m. each evening which invariably contains three little words my husband has dictated: "on my way."

To which I promptly respond, "k".

I now realize that I tend to intertwine my own identity with the "what I do" instead of "who I am".

I distinctly remember having a very hard time adjusting to my new role as a mother when Kaitlyn was born. Although I adored motherhood, I had not anticipated the sudden change in my body or my psyche. How did I go from that woman with "moments of glad grace" to a slightly-rounded-somewhat-frumpy mother overnight? What's more, I'm convinced that one of the reasons that I had such a hard time during my daughters' teenage years was that I saw that very identity, which I had worked so hard to accept, slipping away from me. I became a bereft woman with no visible reason for her roundedness.

Then, with my church lady job, I gained a new identity and threw myself whole-heartedly into that new persona; a strange combination of an NFL defensive player and Mother Teresa. What's more, if you looked past the petite frame of Mother Teresa, I still looked mighty good compared to that football player.

Now this identity was being stripped away from me. If I wasn't an undone mother or a praying juggler, what was I? Who was I going to be now that my work clothes had been donated or stuffed away in cardboard boxes?

I still have to work very hard each day to not adopt the persona of a sick lady. When your world turns you upside down and your very body turns you inside out, it is easy to let yourself fall into the role of invalid. When you spend your days hobbling from one doctor's appointment to the next, you begin to associate yourself with your illness. When you find yourself researching your disease and posting on support groups sites, there is a strong tendency to think that you and your illness are one.

They are not.

You would not have a full understanding of my true emotional state at this time if I did not tell you about an additional sub-plot which was simultaneously unfolding in my life. A few months prior to the onset of my symptoms, my father was moved to a nursing home. He had been diagnosed with Alzheimer's a number of years earlier and it had reached the point that, even with the occasional caregiver, my mother could no longer take care of him at home. Thanks (did I just say "thanks"???) to my illness, I now had the time to accompany my mother on her daily visits to him.

I do not know if you have ever had the honor of being among a group of individuals with dementia, but it can be both heartbreaking and heartwarming at the same time. The things which break your heart are obvious; those which warm your heart are subtle and silent.

I tell you this so that you can understand how I was able to avoid falling into the sick lady syndrome. Quite the opposite, I was able to adroitly jump over that abyss and found myself with a new identity in the role of caregiver; mothering my parents so to speak. My father has since passed away, but I remain convinced that I was placed exactly where I needed to be at the time. My illness and resulting new-found joblessness allowed me to help share the burden with my mother and get to understand and love my father at the very core of his being. I may no longer have been able to manage a large parish community, but I was able to help manage my father's illness.

And since he's gone? I admit I've been floundering a bit since then. It is a good thing that I tend to be quiescent and reflective by nature, for if not this identity theft would be harder to bear.

The Greek philosopher Heraclitis is quoted as saying: "No man ever steps in the same river twice, for it's not the same river and he's not the same man." I am clearly not the same woman I was before I was diagnosed. My priorities have changed. I both think and act with different intent.

Allowing Others to Understand

Earlier today I received a new pair of ugly-but-sensible shoes and, as I tried them on for the first time, thought, "What would happen if I let someone spend a day in you?"

I know for a fact the very first thought that would hit you as you stepped in them would be, "What is wrong with my feet this morning? Why are they tingling? Hurting? Squished? Screaming for air? Are they dead?"

And just imagine where it would go from there.

"Holy Crap, my ankles! Why does it hurt to walk? Why won't my knees go down the stairs like they used to? My left shoulder never hurt me before. Why today? Why can't I wrap my fingers around my coffee cup, and how is it that my hand falls asleep as I do? And lifting it to my lips? I'm shaking like my ancient Aunt Helen! Tell me why I am blinking. What is wrong with my freaking eyes? They're painful! I am NOT going to work today. I wouldn't even be able to get in the car to go to the doctor. Flu! I must have the flu. Water! I need water! Something's wrong with my mouth! Is that dog really trying to tell me that she wants me to get off this couch and let her outside again? I can't even walk from the living room to the kitchen. I'm exhausted. My feet are killing me. SOMETHING IS TERRIBLY WRONG WITH THESE SHOES!!!!!"

Yes, my friend. Something is wrong with those shoes which you stepped into this morning. Those are the shoes of Sjogren's Syndrome, and I'd be glad to give them away for even one day.

Like many autoimmune diseases, Sjogren's is often referred to as an invisible illness because, while there may be an internal war raging within my body, there are no outward or visible signs of illness. Can a casual observer perceive how dry my eyes are? Taste the arid environment in my mouth or experience what it is like to swallow food without water? Can you feel my joint, muscle, and nerve pain? Drag your body around with my fatigue? Become benumbed by my neuropathy? Remember to cover up memory deficits?

I ask you: Can you envision what it is like to walk in my shoes?

Take note that I used the word "allow" in the title of this section. I realize now that this word may be at the crux of what this book is all about. It is about education. Awareness. Knowledge of what it feels like to live with a chronic, painful (if invisible) disease. I state that I am not looking for sympathy and so I get none. What I really want is understanding, and I am not quite sure I have attained that.

I realize that much of this has been my fault. I have not always been truthful with others because I carry with me a pre-conceived notion that they will label me a chronic complainer. I know that this is a danger; that it is virtually impossible to discern other people's thoughts, yet I have somehow allowed this very same notion to make me feel guilty for being ill. I have let my fears of what others may think to color the way I define my sickness to them and let my invisible illness be all-too-invisible to others. Or perhaps I am really just afraid that I'm not ill "enough." I actually blush when others ask me how I feel. I brush it off, give an indistinct reply, or deflect the question away from my health.

Yet if I constantly put a happy face on my life, how should I expect people to respond to me? What, exactly, is the right answer to those who ask "How are you feeling?" or better still, "Are you feeling better yet?" Does the average person want to be treated to a litany of my ailments? I think not. I made that mistake very early one Sunday morning when I truly felt like hell and the poor questioner replied, "Well, I'm sorry I asked!"

Is there a way to educate people in a two sentence reply? What is the right way to let them know that I'm not destined to get better? People are used to hearing about others who are sick – but those people tend to get better, or worse, in time. We are wired to believe in a recovery process. Most people don't just linger in a constant state of limbo with a strange sounding disease for the rest of their lives.

Some, I know, think they have the answer to my problems. They think that if I just moved more, or tried to build up more endurance, my fatigue and joint pain would go away. Many believe that if I changed my diet, eliminating gluten or dairy, I would feel better. Some even hint that they, too, have pain like I do. Believe me my friend, if you had experienced the joint pain I have, you and your new shoes would have hobbled to the doctor ages ago.

This very morning I woke up in such pain that an involuntary cry came out of my mouth. Have you ever started your day by sobbing, "Oh no! No! No! No!" Some of you may be unhappy when your alarm clock goes off, but I venture to guess that there are very few of you who are unhappy because you are no longer in that blessed (and often elusive) state where you don't feel the sensation of pain.

I have also come to the conclusion that some may think that I have taken the easy out. I can't help but feel that they have applied a filter to their perceptions of how a sick person should act and I have come up wanting. Have they forgotten that I worked through every hardship and obstacle placed in my way before? Do they understand that I knew I had these antibodies for a full four years before I acknowledged them? Why, then, would they think that I had taken a ticket to a blissful existence of nothingness, neuropathy, and naps?

Yet here is the kicker: As hinted in the introduction to this book, some of those who I most long to speak with about my illness, never ask. I would be lying if I told you that this does not hurt. It does; and I have spent many a tearless night agonizing over this.

I cannot leave you with the impression that no one has been supportive, concerned, or understanding of my plight. As you may have guessed, my daughters have been a huge help to me. My husband, too, has been my rock throughout. And there are other members of my family and a few dear friends who have been very caring and compassionate. I am grateful for them and know I don't thank them nearly as often as I should. And still I find myself grateful for another reason, for my own suffering has opened up a whole new level of awareness. It has made me more empathetic and compassionate. I am now resolved not to make the same mistakes that others around me have made.

Perhaps I have been the one who has, at last, been allowed to understand.

Anxiety and Depression

I thought at first that I would be able to skirt around this topic with characteristic humor, but have subsequently realized that treating anxiety and depression in this manner would not be fair to all those who, like me, suffer from the debilitating effects of these afflictions. I also realized that I have never spoken to anyone in detail about my own depression beyond those who have a nameplate carefully tacked to their door.

Unlike my anxiety and Sjogren's symptoms, it is hard for me to date the onset of my depression. I do recall years back, when my children were in their pre-teen days, sitting on the side of my bed sobbing for hours in the morning after all other occupants had left the house. Why? I honestly don't know. What I do know is that I would eventually pull myself together by taking a shower and forcing myself to get on with my day. At other times that same shower served as my escape, the only place in a crowded house in which I could cry my eyes out.

Did anyone notice? No. Did I let anyone know? Of course not.

Anxiety, on the other hand, was a tad bit more disconcerting for me and proved to be a whole lot harder to hide. Although I had experienced a few panic attacks in my adult years (all involving an inordinate fear of my children drowning) something changed the year that Megan entered high school and Kaitlyn went off to college. These were the days that anxiety slowly and insidiously became my constant companion. Something began happening to me as I drove – always late and in a constant rush. My heart began to flutter, my stomach to tighten, a big hollow feeling would arrive in my chest, my light-headedness causing me to feel as if I were about to pass out. Soon I became afraid to drive and at times even to be a passenger. Highway travel was the worst, for I would envision an accident around every turn or become convinced that my door would suddenly open mid-stream, sucking me out of the car. Never one to be nervous around crowds before, I began to dislike feeling closed in with other humans and standing in front of crowds. I also began to worry about traveling far from home.

It was anxiety and one particular panic attack which finally drove me to mention my condition at one of my dreaded doctor's appointments when they called me in to check my blood pressure. The nurse practitioner offered medication to me. "Are you also depressed?" she asked me.

"No, I don't think so," I replied.

Nevertheless she went on to prescribe an SSRI (Selective Serotonin Reuptake Inhibitor) for me to take everyday and an additional anti-anxiety medication for me to take for situational anxiety. I remember this particular appointment being around my birthday in early October.

It was only after my depression began to lift that I realized that I had been living under its yoke all along. I distinctly remember standing in a bakery on a day in late November, feeling happy. This was the first time I could actually lay claim to feeling joy in as long as I could remember. I thought to myself, "Here I am, standing in a line in the bakery waiting to buy turkey cookies and I think I just may be happy! I am not sad at any rate, ergo I must be happy!"

Three years later, when Megan went off to college, I mistakenly believed that I no longer needed to take medication and proceeded to wean myself off, yet still taking quick-acting anti-anxiety pills whenever I experienced what I termed "situational anxiety". An agonizing four years later I was such a mess that I was forced to return to medication and therapy.

This book is not meant to be about my experiences with depression and anxiety so I will not bore you with a host of agonizing stories – like the time I was trapped in a parking lot for a half-hour during the height of the Christmas shopping season afraid to back out of my parking place for fear of hitting a pedestrian, or the time I drove my daughter to a doctor's appointment over the Tappan Zee Bridge and couldn't bring myself to drive back. Nor will I tell you about the countless times I would enter the bathroom at a family party, begin to cry, and then be forced to slap water on my face and shore myself up for my reemergence.

I will, however, tell you about the New Year's Eve which forced me to begin to see a therapist and return to medication. Leah, who was lovingly nicknamed Ponzi at this time, was leaving the following day for a college class in Sweden. She had turned 21 just two days earlier and, up to this point, both her mind and energies had been devoted to a three-day birthday bash in New York City. She returned home on New Year's Eve exhausted, hung over, and just a tad bit cranky; not a single thing packed for her month-long trip. Not only that, she needed to purchase numerous supplies, one of them being a long warm coat which would cover her tush as she sat on the frozen stools at those famous ice bars.

Now it seems to be an unwritten law of nature that no matter where the unpleasantries in a household are coming from, it is clearly the mother's fault. Why deal with the actual source of the problem when you can blame it on an innocent bystander? What's more, the innocent bystander was the one who had to wake the merrymaker from her hangover nap and drag her to the dreaded mall to purchase the coat. After the long and arduous process of buying two coats, Leah ran through the mall to get a few more essentials while I sat in the car.

Anxious. Desperate. Depressed. Not a single anti-anxiety pill on hand to help me through.

By the time we were ready to leave the mall it was dark and my problem with nighttime driving only exacerbated my panic. (The thought of sitting in the passenger seat while a hung-over-sleep-deprived daughter drove was immediately ruled out.) I drove to the next stop with my hands gripped tightly around the steering wheel – wildly fighting the impulse to swerve the car and drive off the road in one fell swoop. I waited for Leah to leave the car and enter the pharmacy before I lost it. She returned to the car ten minutes later to find her mother in a state in which she had never seen her before. I continued to sob uncontrollably for another ten minutes before I could collect myself enough to start the car. What's worse, we were due to stop at my sister's house for a glass of wine to celebrate the start of the New Year. Knowing that once home I may never leave the house again, I opted not to stop and pick up my husband.

Upon entering my sister's front door, my zombie-like body immediately guided me to that now-familiar bathroom from which I reemerged like a jovial changeling, mumbled a lame excuse to explain the absence of the man I left at home, chugged my first glass of wine like it was an infusion meant to restore my very lifeblood, and proceeded to chat away cheerfully as if I were the hostess of the television New Year's Eve countdown.

Leah was both flabbergasted and frightened – so much so, that on her way to the airport the next day she contacted a therapist she knew and asked her to call me. I am forever grateful to her that she did.

I suppose that I should consider myself lucky that I was already on medication when I became ill, for depression is often a byproduct of living with chronic illness. The trauma brought on by pain, uncertainty, change of lifestyle, fatigue, and shifting relationships is sometimes more than even the most-grounded among us can handle. Adding the effects of depression to a lifelong illness can prove to be devastating.

Keep in mind that the symptoms of depression are often as insidious and indiscriminate as those of my autoimmune disease. They are, by nature, creepers – sneaking up on a unsuspecting victim without notice or fanfare, until in time you find yourself living alongside them like part of your extended family – kissing cousins, so to speak.

I can sense that my depression is slowly deepening as I attempt to live within the tempest of an unremitting illness. I am aware of a veil gradually descending over my life. I clearly sense a loss of confidence in myself, as that identity theft leaves me unable to lay claim to positive feedback and the feeling of camaraderie that I received from work. I have lost the ability to make small talk with those who I would classify as acquaintances, and find I've become distant with many family members as well. The growing sense of isolation I feel may sometimes appear to be of my own making, yet much of it is what I view as reactionary.

Sjogren's is often described as a disease of flares but, in reality, I experience flares of despondency as well. A person with persistent depressive disorder will also experience major depressive episodes. In the two years since becoming ill my world has come hurdling down upon me on a handful of occasions. And let me tell you honestly, I would much rather deal with the physical pain that my illness brings than the utter despair, desolation, hopelessness, and panic that one of these episodes brings.

Part Three: Thriving with Autoimmunity

16. The Mind-Body Connection

So be sure when you step, step with care and great tact,
and remember that life is a great balancing act.
— *Dr. Seuss*

By now you may be a bit depressed yourself – picturing your now-favorite author stuck in a quagmire from which there is no escape. Let us return for a moment to that author's distressed cinematic queries which opened this book:

She inclines her head towards heaven and asks, "How on earth did it get to be like this? My children sick? My own life forever altered by an unceasing illness? Walling myself off from my husband? Becoming isolated from family and friends? And when, dear Lord, when will things get better? Please tell me when!"

Please note that there was no inquiry into when things would be perfect, or ideal, or returned to a pre-sickness state. We have learned that these autoimmune diseases and conditions are not reversible or curable. We know that we can mask some symptoms, ease some pain, and – in some cases – even hope to slow the progress of the disease. So the only question one can rightfully ask in my situation is, "When will things become more bearable?"

Or perhaps, "How can I better accept these things?"

The first obligation a person in my situation has is to be sure she is getting the best possible medical care available. The next reasonable obligation is to make sure that the emotional toll brought about by the disease(s) does not begin to dominate her life.

And this, my friends, is where the triumvirate of *Mind, Body, and Spirit* come into play.

The Problem of Perception

Did you know that scientists estimate that we have over 37 trillion cells working in our bodies? When you think about staggering numbers like that, it is only natural to assume that our bodies must have complete control over our health and wellbeing.

Think about it. I am with my body every day; attached more closely than I am to my husband, and I don't recall ever taking any vows with it. There was no "to have to and hold, in sickness and in health" pledge in our relationship. But still, I live in its skin, let its lungs breathe my air, and allow its heart to send my lifeblood flowing through me. What's more, I suffer through its aches, shuffle on its feet, and endure the sabulous dryness it has brought to me.

When first diagnosed I became absolutely convinced that I had been betrayed by my body. I have since realized that this reaction came about precisely because the language surrounding autoimmune diseases is often quite harsh and invariably evokes a feeling of treachery. And an autoimmuner like me reads or hears such language all of the time. I challenge you to research any autoimmune disease and not find the words "attack" or "destroy" within the first five sentences. Researchers may not understand the "whys" or "hows" behind each disease but the evidence is clear: Autoimmune diseases occur when the fighter cells in your body begin to mistake healthy tissue for an intruder and start to turn against the very organs they were designed to protect.

How would you expect an individual to feel when they discover that their body has turned on itself? Disappointed. Betrayed. Abnormal. I admit I felt all of these.

My joints weren't hurting because I had caught a virus. My eyes were not dry because of an infection. I couldn't even blame my fatigue on a deadly invader like cancer. No. I felt sick simply because my body was destroying itself for no known reason. And every time I tried to learn more about this disease called Sjogren's Syndrome, those thoughts were reinforced in my brain. At times I even thought to myself, "How could my body be so dumb?"

Why was it turning on itself?

Yet somehow in the first months of my I-can-live-with-this mania which followed my diagnosis, I stumbled upon a few things which helped me approach my illness from a different perspective. I learned to take a step back and look for hope, gratitude, and joy in any situation. I also discovered that I have no reason to despise my illness.

It dawned on me that my physical presence is not all there is to me. Those three little pounds of gray matter that I call my brain produce 70,000 thoughts per day. What if I employed those thoughts to help with my healing and acceptance?

What if I focused on the positives instead of getting discouraged by the negatives? I don't always have to be happy; but I can be joyful. I have a soul, energy flows, and a Zen garden. I have peace working within me. I don't think that any of the above would enter the census in a cell count, but they are on my side. I now know that my body must feel my pain too. And so I have tried to find a way to bring mind, body, and spirit together to make this better for all of us – as well as for those trillions of cells.

Although I may be struggling with identity theft – not quite knowing who I am at the present time – I have no problem knowing who I am not, and I am confident that I am not a PhD, brain surgeon, psychologist, nutritionist, the Dalai Lama, Tai Chi master, Luke Skywalker, yogi, the Pope, or certified life coach.

The information I offer here and in the following chapters is not intended to be medical advice, but rather information acquired by reading reference books, careful research on the internet, and my personal experiences of living with an autoimmune disease. These are tips which I feel are helpful for living a healthy lifestyle and acquiring an appropriate mindset to battle the effects of autoimmunity. Please remember that these tips are meant to be used in combination with traditional medical treatments, not in place of them. All of them are intended to do no harm when united with Western medical approaches, but all should be discussed, and approved, by a physician before undertaking them.

There is, however, one exception to that rule. I would never enter a physician's office and ask permission to follow my suggestion of "forest bathing." I think it is safe to say that all of us can attempt that little tip without prior approval by anyone in the medical community.

Attitude of Gratitude

Because, as we have discovered, I am often "Zenchanted," shortly after being diagnosed I sought out the Center for Well Being sponsored by our local hospital. This center offers both integrative and complementary medical approaches, along with yoga, meditation, tai chi, and stress reduction classes. After failing miserably in a restorative yoga class (let's just say my proclivity for vertigo got the better of me and instead of the pose, *Downward Facing Dog*, I ended up in *Woman with Face in Toilet Bowl*) I enrolled in a tai chi class. During my second class, as we were warming up, I made a remark something akin to the following: "My stupid ankle won't do that." My careless statement was enough for the instructor to stop the class and remind us all that, no matter our deficiencies, we need to be thankful for all that our bodies do for us each day.

What an awakening! I had been consumed with all of the negatives surrounding my condition and forgot to be grateful for the positives. My body wasn't abandoning me. Imagine all of the systems which were still working in perfect order. My heart was still beating umpteen times per minute, my lungs were certainly exchanging carbon dioxide for oxygen, and my body was getting the nutrients it needed. I was walking, talking, thinking, speaking, hearing, and seeing.

What should I be, if not thankful?

That philosophy has been the very one that has saved me.

The practice of tai chi, as it turns out, is not simply a series of physical movements; it is a mental discipline as well. It is a life practice which involves acquiring a mindset of healing, peace, energy, gratefulness, and love towards ourselves and others. At the conclusion of each class our instructor ends with the words, "And we are grateful for our abundance and our blessings."

Yes I am!

Stress "Out"

It is a proven fact that the physiological effects of stress can trigger a flare of symptoms in many autoimmune diseases. The "fight or flight" response ingrained in us from primitive days still springs up in our reactions to stress. This stress response, which proved to be a lifesaver for cavemen, is just not productive for us today.

Let us return to the months prior to the onset of my symptoms. It began when my mother had a recurrence of breast cancer which involved first a lumpectomy, and then a mastectomy. No sooner had my mother recovered than my father suffered a stroke and, after a stint in the ICU, ended up a permanent resident in a nursing home. Leah's illness arrived next on the scene, bringing with it a barrage of doctors' visits and a steady stream of worry and uncertainty. Megan's disease markers rose.

And although these other stressors may seem minor in comparison, we need to consider my ill-timed fall down the stairs brought about by the addition of the foster puppy from hell and the prolonged hospice care of the family cat who eventually went to cat heaven. I then had to explain to my daughters why I opted for the $50 group cremation for that cat (now sadly dubbed Lymphoma Mayzie) instead of the $250 individual one.

Those girls wanted her ashes.

Then there were the pressures attached to my job as church lady. I would typically work six (and sometimes seven) days a week. And even when I was not technically working on a Sunday, a trip to church with the intent to worship always turned into an occupational event – as toilets clogged, microphones malfunctioned, and steam-heated boiler pipes leaked. Parishioners who spied me immediately thought it the ideal time to lodge a complaint or relay important scheduling information. I would return home from church services a human bulletin board; sticky notes hanging from every available appendage of my body.

When you consider all of these factors, is it any wonder I came down with the flu for the first time in my adult life? I remain convinced that the flu and the stress preceding it were the triggers which set my disease into full swing.

But how can I eliminate stress from my life now so I can be as healthy as possible? In truth, eliminating the pressures inherent with my job has reduced my anxiety level and left me time for meditation, prayer, and stillness. Yet other worries remain and are unavoidable. The death of my father, care of my mother, and unease over my family's health still continue to take a toll on me; but at least I am calm once again and do not feel as if I am caught in an eddy of chaotic happenings.

Meditation

When it comes to bringing mind and body together, meditation is clearly an ideal therapeutic tool. There have been thousands of studies performed on the impact of meditation on health and well-being. Meditation has been found to lower high blood pressure, increase serotonin production, improve the immune system, increase energy levels, decrease tension-related pain, reduce depression and anxiety, increase focus, and promote a general sense of well-being. What's more, studies show that these benefits come after practicing meditation for just 20 minutes a day for as little as six weeks.

There are dozens of meditation methods and techniques to choose from. Most of them involve a focus on breathing, a mantra, or word. A few, like chi quong, are moving meditations. Some are done using beads along with repetitive prayers or mantras. Some are practiced in specific stance or poses. Others can be practiced from your living room couch or your favorite easy chair. A few, like Tibetan singing bowls use sound and vibration to restore balance.

I try to practice a Christian type of meditation, called Centering Prayer, which flows from the contemplative tradition of Christianity. The goal of this method is to detach yourself from the stream of everyday thought, allowing your mind to become empty so that you are available to hear what God wants to convey. "Be still and know that I am God" (Psalm 46). Before beginning the practice, you choose one word which then becomes your center. When your mind begins to stray and everyday thoughts intrude, you gently return to your word to remind you to empty your mind again.

This method of prayer and meditation makes perfect sense to me. If prayer is, by definition, a dialogue with God, the one-way communication that most of us have simply does not seem to be logical. How can God respond to us if we are busy doing all of the talking? I am sure we have all had the misfortune of accepting a dinner invitation with an acquaintance who talked only of him/herself all evening. Of course God's response is never in formed words and it is God, not we, who directs the message according to our needs. His response may come in a wise decision later in the day, inkling later in the week, or simply in a feeling of serenity when needed most.

Is it difficult to get all of the pieces just right? To slow down a mind which seems determined to break an Olympic speed record? While I am sometimes able to drop into a meditative state easily, at other times I spend 18 of my 20 minutes battling interfering thoughts. But the sense of contentment received in those two remaining minutes is enough for me.

I beg you not to let my interpretation of this ancient Christian practice stand as your only instruction. For those interested in finding out more about centering prayer, I encourage you to read *Open Mind, Open Heart* by Thomas Keating, a Cistercian monk in the Benedictine tradition.

Any type of meditation can leave us with the same feeling. Just this evening, as I sat down, I could feel the softness of my living room couch which has, at times, become an enemy and symbol of my illness; but suddenly it was different. My pains and aches melted away, absorbed in the gentle feel of the pillows of the sofa. With Giardia Jax resting on the edge at my shoulder and the ever-loving Kasey at my feet, I suddenly had an overwhelming feeling of contentment. My body felt lifted, lighter.

Through meditation I am reminded to take those moments of serenity and gratification and carry them forth into the rest of my life, hoping they will sustain me during more difficult times.

Mindfulness Matters

The ability to benefit by paying this sort of attention to my present surroundings has come about through another type of meditation. I now incorporate short, mindfulness breaks throughout the day. Certainly no expert on mindfulness, I rely instead on an app which provides short, two-minute morning and night guided meditations. I have also chosen to set reminders to take 30-second pauses throughout the day.

The practice of mindfulness, which springs in most part from teachings of the Buddha, has been described as the nonjudgmental awareness of experiences in the present moment. The effort is to not intentionally add anything to our present experience, but simply to be aware of what is going on without losing ourselves in anything that arises.

Not surprisingly, it is the nonjudgmental part of this practice which is the hardest for me to accept. For instance, one of the quick reminders during the day reads, "Can you feel your toes?" Imagine how hard it is for a person with neuropathy to leave their negative emotions regarding the answer to that question out of the equation. On the flip side, when it comes to performing a body scan, I often note that I have produced more saliva, which often happens while I am in a calm state, but I try to remain impartial about this as well.

As with any type of meditation, the more you practice mindfulness, the more benefits you will receive from it. I have also learned to use mindfulness practices to help me deal with my anxiety; replacing anxiety medication with meditation. As I feel the first physiologic signs of panic hit, instead of reaching for that little pill, I now try to employ mindfulness practices to simply BE with those feelings. I have learned that much of my anxiety is anticipatory, not wanting to experience the physical discomfort associated with a panic attack. Yet, if I am in a time and place when I am able to sit with this discomfort in non-judgmental awareness, the feeling will often dissipate.

Similarly, mindfulness practices can also help us deal with chronic suffering. In this context we need to differentiate between pain and suffering in the Buddhist tradition. Pain is a sensation we feel in our bodies – a sensation we have no control over. Suffering is what comes about from attaching negative feelings to that pain, seeking avoidance of it. As is often said, "Pain is inevitable; suffering is not." With mindfulness practices we can learn to sit with our pain, to know it, and almost to welcome it. Although the pain will not dissipate, our suffering often will.

17. Honor Thy Body

If you never did, you should.
These things are fun and fun is good!

– Dr. Seuss

You Are What You Eat

Clearly I am not the ideal author for this topic; for if you were to judge an individual by this maxim, I am macaroni and cheese.

The hallmark reaction of any rheumatic disease is inflammation, and so it follows that the best protection is to be on an anti-inflammatory diet. An anti-inflammatory diet is one rich in whole grains, fruits, and vegetables. Processed foods are never good and should be avoided at all costs. Many researchers believe that sensitivity to gluten or nightshade vegetables may contribute to autoimmune reactions. Others believe that fasting can help overcome the autoimmune process. Some studies have also shown that eating a vegan diet without any animal products helps to control inflammation as well. I urge you to discuss your diet with your doctor or nutritionist and then take a walk through any bookstore, spy the vast array of cookbooks dedicated to autoimmune diets, and find one that is right for you.

I was a vegetarian for over two years but have since returned to the chicken-and-turkey-eating realm. I have recently added salmon to my diet because it is rich in omega 3 fatty acids which also help to stop inflammation in the body. And I now try to limit my gluten intake to whole grains only, and try desperately to eat more berries and nuts.

Lest I give you a false impression, I need to confess that I am still a certified carb-a-holic whose only wish is to be swimming in an ocean of cheese. To add insult to injury, some of the foods that I most love are the hardest for me to swallow. I can't tell you the number of times I have nearly choked on a bagel or simple cracker. How can I even explain to you the agony I now feel when I have to forego the sample cheese selections on those little toothpicks in the grocery store because that free chunk of cheesy-heaven will cause me to buy a two dollar bottle of spring water or will be stuck in my throat until I run outside and reach the bottle of water I so carelessly left in my car?

My daughters, on the other hand, do not follow my example.

Kaitlyn has been a vegetarian for over ten years. She also eats no dairy and limits her intake of carbohydrates and gluten. She believes that her diet helps to keep her symptoms in check. The fact that she was able to train for, and run, a half-marathon may just be proof-positive that she is on the right track.

Megan has been a vegetarian for almost as long as Kaitlyn and has, from time to time, adopted a dairy and gluten free diet but has not quite felt the benefits that her sister has when attempting a vegan diet.

Leah had a three year stint as a vegetarian but now eats chicken, turkey, and fish. Unlike me, Leah is a firm believer in juicing and, again, rarely eats any thing containing gluten.

Even though Kaitlyn no longer lives at home, I believe it would be hard to find another household in America consuming more vegetables and fruits than mine. Do you know how many bags of kale and stalks of celery it takes to make one little juice drink? And how about my husband's blender drink each morning filled with kale, spinach, cucumbers, carrots, chia and flax seeds, and topped off with vegan protein powder? Megan's breakfast of avocado, almonds, and hot sauce? Last night's dinner table alone sported grilled chicken along with a medley of grilled asparagus, onions, peppers, zucchini, and mushrooms. Add to that snow peas and sliced tomato with fresh basil. Oh yes, and a spoonful or two of brown rice left over from the night before.

I toyed with the vegetables and ate the chicken and rice.

Nutritional Supplements

I may have a tough time sticking to an anti-inflammatory diet yet find no problem in taking supplements or adding anti-inflammatory herbs and spices to my diet. It is encouraging to find that almost all of the supplements I now take have been suggested or prescribed to me by my physicians, a sign that the medical community recognizes the beneficial effects of certain medical foods and vitamins. Beyond a generic multivitamin I add the following:

> **Vitamin D3** – When first tested, my vitamin D level was on the border of a major vitamin D deficiency, which can contribute to joint pain and fatigue. Keep in mind, natural sunlight is a major source of vitamin D and I cannot spend any time in the sun.

Calcium – Along with vitamin D, I take a prescription calcium supplement each day. The steroid, prednisone, often drains calcium from your body and D3 needs to be present to break down the calcium you ingest.

Omega 3 Fish Oil – Beyond its well-known benefits for heart health, Omega 3 fatty acids promote eye health and help regulate immune and inflammatory responses.

Biotin – Helps to strengthen hair and nails and to slow down hair loss, a side effect of many immunosuppressants.

L-Methylfolate and Folic Acid – Prescription folic acid is used to offset side effects from certain immunosuppressants. L-Methylfolate is a particular form of folic acid that is already activated and ready for the body to use. Studies have shown that up to 70 percent of patients with depression have problems processing folic acid and so it is prescribed along with my anti-depressant. Interestingly enough, L-Methylfolate has also been prescribed for my peripheral neuropathy along with the following.

Vitamin B6, B12, and Alpha Lipoic Acid – All three of these supplements are thought to help with peripheral neuropathy. Once again, I take a prescription supplement of the activated form of vitamins B6 and 12 and an over-the-counter form of alpha lipoic acid.

Magnesium – I take a magnesium supplement to help with blood pressure, heart health, and muscle cramping. Research has shown that those who take proton pump inhibitors to reduce the symptoms of GERD may have low levels of magnesium.

Tumeric, Ginger, and Cinnamon – There are claims that these spices have anti-inflammatory properties and reduce joint pain and so I add them to any soup, stews, or rubs I can.

Green Tea – The anti-inflammatory benefits of drinking green tea have been widely touted and I drink at least two cups each day.

Be sure to inform your doctors of all supplements you are taking, as some may affect how different medications are absorbed by your body.

Moving Muscles

I have always been a couch potato, yet every doctor, book, and website will tell you that moving aching joints and muscles will help to alleviate pain and fatigue. And so I tried.

In the first months of my illness, I joined the local YMCA in order to take part in the Arthritis Foundation's water aerobics classes. This gentle and non-weight bearing exercise was perfect for me (along with the host of 90-year-olds who were in the class with me.) When the schedule changed and these classes were moved to the 9:00 a.m. time slot, I stopped participating. I am no longer a morning person.

I then tried participating in full-blown water aerobics classes later in the day, dialing down the level of activity to what I felt was right for me, but was hit with *The Walking Dead Wipeout* once too often for my tastes. And because my feet were not on terra firma while walking in the pool, I experienced the additive bonus of motion sickness. Many was the day I left that gym unsure if I would make it home without pulling over to the side of the road to employ my *Woman with Face in Toilet Bowl* position.

But do not take my own story as typical.

Despite the swelling and aching she experiences on a daily basis, Kaitlyn pushes through her pain regularly to exercise, run, and work out. Yes, the discomfort that first appeared on that high school lacrosse field was still with her when she successfully ran that half-marathon four years ago, but Kaitlyn believes that this level of exercise helps to ease the pain which comes with her spondyloarthropathy and keeps her mentally and emotionally healthy.

Leah, too, tries to be an avid exerciser; although muscle weakness has relegated her to physical therapy sessions, yoga, and simple walking for the time being.

Circulating Energy

The form of exercise which has come to my rescue is the practice of tai chi, a calming series of movements performed in a prescribed sequence. Originally from China and considered a form of martial arts, the particular type of tai chi I practice is Wu style tai chi – a grateful and healing-based approach to core energy circulation and movement. The very words "tai chi" translate to "supreme ultimate," but the "chi" (or "qi") is considered to mean "that which gives life" or simply, the life-giving energy that flows within you.

The practice of tai chi has been found to help with balance, coordination, muscle strength, flexibility, mental and physical discipline. Often described as "meditation in motion," tai chi can also be referred to as "medication in motion". It can lower blood pressure, reduce inflammation, and decrease levels of depression. One study even found that practicing tai chi increases the ability and speed by which the nerves send signals back to the brain, therefore helping with peripheral neuropathy.

Tai chi is by no means the only discipline which centers on the body's ability to move and circulate the energy (chi or qi) as a mechanism for healing. I have also participated in chi quong and tai chi chih® classes. Breathing, circulation, and energy centers are fundamental to all three of these disciplines.

The practice of chi quong centers on breath work and movement together – supplying oxygen to the body so that, in theory, diseased energies cannot thrive. My tai chi instructor devotes a portion of our tai chi classes to the practice of chi quong, as do I with my own personal practice. I have also attended hour-long sessions of chi quong offered at my local hospital.

While a more modern practice, tai chi chih® (Joy through Movement) is a moving meditation which consists of 19 movements and one pose and helps to improve health, creativity, performance, and intuition. I find the repetitive movements of tai chi chih to be both soothing and energizing – truly a meditation for me.

Vibrational Healing

Approximately once a month I attend a Tibetan singing bowl meditation. The vibration and tones emitted by the bowls are used to cleanse and balance the body's chakras. I suppose anyone who has stuck out a yoga class longer than I knows that both the Hindu and Buddhist traditions teach that there are seven major chakras in the body. Each is envisioned as a swirling wheel within the core of your body and stores a different kind of energy. This energy, called "prana", keeps us vibrant, healthy, and alive. Conversely, blocked chakras are believed to create illness.

At a singing bowl meditation the practitioner invites different notes from the bowls, each corresponding with one of the body's chakras, by rubbing a mallet around the rim or striking the side of the bowl. When used for healing, the bowls are often placed on the body of the receiver. Nothing can prepare you for the energy felt within your entire body when a whorling bowl is placed on your stomach or your ears are filled with the vibrational tones of a bowl placed near your head. At times you can almost breathe in the very vibration. Regardless of whether you personally believe that wheels called chakras exist in your body, it is both healing and cleansing to let your mind drift along with the sound the bowls emit.

It may sound to you like I am mixing my metaphors. How can I take part in disciplines centered around both "chi" and "prana"? Why do I have Tibetan bowls playing in the background while employing a Christian method of meditation? Gregorian chant while practicing tai chi? The answer is simple. Just like everything else in the universe, we are beings of energy and vibration – and I believe in positive energy, no matter where others believe it springs from or whatever they choose to call it. I trust that all energy comes from the same Source and is sustained and nourished by the same Spirit. I also know for sure that even when I drag myself against my will to any class or meditation, I emerge refreshed, energized, grateful, and happy to have shared time with like-minded people.

Needles, Hands, and Meridians

There are many additional modalities which employ, channel, or direct these energy flows in order to provide healing. Acupuncture, jin shin jyutsu, reiki, and healing touch are those which come to mind.

In my quest to restore energy and relieve my symptoms of joint pain and neuropathy, I have turned to reiki, jin shin jyutsu, and acupuncture. Although some may be skeptical about the efficacy of these methods, I have found each of them to be helpful in their own way.

Just as we spoke about charkas in connection with singing bowl meditations, the practice of reiki also concentrates on balancing or cleansing these seven charkas (which store vital life energy) in order to activate the natural healing processes in the patient's body and restore physical and emotional well-being. While there may not be any one "typical" reiki experience, before a session the practitioner may ask the client what they wish to achieve from the session (once again using the client's thoughts and the mind/body connection to take part in the healing.) After setting an intention for the session, the practitioner's hands then move through specific hand positions – usually hovering just above the patient's body, but at times employing light touch as well. A client may experience a feeling of warmth during the session or simply fall into a state of welcome relaxation.

The Touch of Healing by Alice Burmeister is considered the authoritative guidebook for the practice of jin shin jyutsu, a time-honored method of healing in the Japanese tradition. Jin shin balances your body's energy by using the practitioner's fingers and hands to eliminate stress, create emotional equilibrium, and relieve pain. Once again, the practice centers on the energy pathways in your body and the 26 sites where this energy is concentrated. When imbalances block these pathways – resulting in pain, illness, stress, or emotional turmoil – placement of fingers on these particular sites along the pathways allow the practitioner (or the patient themselves) to release vital energy flows and restore proper energy circulation.

Within two minutes of the start of my first jin shin treatment, tears began to roll down my face. To this day, I am sure the practitioner remains convinced that the sudden flow of tears was due to the unblocking of the pathways to my tear glands, and in all likelihood it was. I have been embarrassed to tell her, however, that she unblocked a different sort of pathway in that first session as well; an emotional one. Newly diagnosed, I had been poked, prodded, and prescribed by every healthcare professional I had met along the way. Add to that the fact that I still carried with me the mindset that my body had turned on itself, and I was a physical and emotional wreck.

This was the first time since being diagnosed that anyone had touched my body with the intent to heal. Her hands were warm, practiced, and curative and her mere touch caused me to weep like an injured child whose mother had just kissed her wound. Since that time I have benefited from many jin shin jyutsu sessions with the same practitioner. All have proved to be restorative and healing.

This should serve as a lesson for all in the healthcare industry, as well those of us who suffer, or love those who suffer, from chronic pain. Let us never again underestimate the therapeutic nature of touch. In fact, our local hospital now provides jin shin practitioners who, when requested, visit patients' bedsides. Reiki sessions are also conducted on site in the cancer center. Healing touch is now being offered to patients who are undergoing chemotherapy or other infusion treatments.

Now allow me touch on acupuncture.

From the Latin "acus" (needle) and the English word "puncture" the ancient practice of acupuncture is a key component of Traditional Chinese Medicine. It is a technique in which practitioners stimulate specific points on the body – most often by inserting thin needles through the skin. These needles stimulate the flow of vital energy or "Qi" (pronounced "chi") along the meridians or energy pathways of the body.

But does acupuncture work? Results from a number of studies suggest that acupuncture may help ease types of pain that are often chronic such as low-back pain, neck pain, and knee pain. The National Institute of Health says, "Acupuncture appears to be a reasonable option for people with chronic pain to consider."

When I had my first appointment with an acupuncture

practitioner at my local hospital's Center for Well Being, he asked me to tell him which areas were problematic for me.

"Everywhere" I replied.

Upon reflection, I am quite sure that he didn't have enough needles in his kit for the response of "everywhere" and so we decided to settle on two things which were bothering me most that day. And then he went to work. Because the *Pain Train* had decided on an extended stay in my left pinkie, he inserted a few needles in my head (which appears to be the treasure map to many other parts of my body) and then asked me to check my finger. No pain. Another half-dozen or so in my ankles and chest, and he left the room for 30 minutes in order for me to rest and restore my energy flow. And flow it did! I was not prepared to experience those first few minutes spent lying down in that healing atmosphere with an unknown number of needles stuck in my body. I felt energy (or blood, who knows) buzzing through my body at lightning speed, bringing vigor to each and every body part. This was the direct opposite of *The Pain Train!* This was a true sense of my body healing itself, temporary though it may have been.

After that we often concentrated on the neuropathy in my hands and feet. Believe it or not, the treasure map still pointed to my head, and so he inserted about a dozen needles there. One day I arrived with neck pain and the map pointed to my ears instead. All I know is that I arrived at each session with a heavy, leaden feeling and emerged feeling lighter and less painful.

I feel the need to add a bit of a disclaimer here. Visiting with an acupuncturist is not for the faint of heart – not only because your body will be used like a pin cushion – but because of the personal nature of questions you will need to answer. If you do not feel comfortable speaking about the quality and quantity of what you eliminate from your body, perhaps you should stay at home in your bathroom for – like a ruler in medieval times – it may seem as if your Royal Tailor has suddenly felt the urge to act as your personal Groom of the Stool.

And one more thing. Take extra care before visiting to make sure your belly button does not have any lint or fuzzies in it, lest they somehow get sewn in there for good.

Enough said.

Nurturing Your Senses

Perhaps you don't have the means to attend a tai chi class or you live in an area where acupuncture or meditation classes are not available. Complementary medical approaches are often expensive and not covered by insurance. Once again, I stress that all traditional medical approaches, as prescribed by specialists in the appropriate field, should be followed and adhered to. I list here other, low-cost and easy methods we can use to awaken our senses, ease our pain, and lift our spirits. None of the methods listed below will interfere with traditional medicine and can only enhance our experience of a holistic approach to healing:

> **Nurture your sense of smell**. I have worn a certain perfume for years which is meant to evoke the smell of the Irish Sea. I discovered long ago that this simple aroma makes me feel good. Years ago, before I even knew that I suffered from depression, I would often lie

in bed at night, sniffing my wrist and think, "At least I have this smell to keep me going." This was my first experience with aromatherapy before I knew what the word meant. Almost every health food store now sells chakra sprays, natural candles, and essential oils. While seasonal paraffin candles may smell good, it is my humble opinion that the aroma of things found in nature like jasmine, lavender, and peppermint do more to lift my spirits than a candle whose fragrance was carefully crafted in a chemistry lab.

Nurture your sense of touch. Use the Jin Shin Jyutsu method of patiently holding each finger in turn. Just as with reflexology, many eastern modalities believe that different parts of our fingers correspond to different emotions and organs in our bodies. Holding your thumb, for instance, is believed to be good for an upset stomach or to lessen anxiety. You can also give yourself a hand massage. Be sure to massage your palm, just a little closer to your thumb first, to activate the minor hand chakra which allows you to become open to the healing touch of massage. Become familiar with the stress relief and energy flows which are believed to come from holding your fingers and hands in Buddhist or Hindu Mudras. Massage your head and temple area, taking special note of the feeling invoked as you lovingly touch the area where the center of your forehead meets your hairline. There is a reason that the foreheads of monarchs, prophets, and those who are ill are anointed there with precious oil.

Nurture your sense of sound. Take to heart the saying that, "Music calms the savage beast." Do you remember when I spoke of the "puppy from hell" we fostered for two months in our home? I quickly discovered that the only way to calm that crazy canine was to play tranquil music. Classical, new age, chant, and haunting Celtic melodies were her (and my) favorites. On the flip side, upbeat music and familiar tunes can make one happy and excited.

Nurture your sense of sight. Surround yourself with your favorite color. Look – I mean really look – at things around you. Stare at a candle flame as it flickers. Watch another person smile. Notice the raindrops on the windowpane, your cat as he sleeps. We are happiest when we are surrounded by sights that make us happy.

Nurture the innate longing all of us have for nature. Even if you can't take long walks in the woods, bring nature indoors using plants, water, sea shells, and stones which root us to the earth and make us feel grounded. A few stalks of bamboo in a vase of water costs less than ten dollars but allows another living, breathing entity to share our space with us. If you have the chance, transform yourself into a tree hugger. Simply place your hands around six inches from a tree or bush. Notice, and absorb, the positive energy emitted. We are intended to have a synergistic relationship with all plants. A study in Japan found that "forest bathing" is good for you. This Japanese practice of simply being around trees has been shown to lower heart rate and blood pressure, reduce stress hormone production, and improve overall feeling of wellbeing.

Nurture your sense of creativity. Begin to paint, journal, or play a musical instrument. Did you know it has been found that the confessional nature of memoirs makes writing them a potentially powerful tool for healing?

Immerse your senses in water. Approximately 60 percent of the adult human body is comprised of water. Is it any wonder that we are, by nature, drawn to the sound, sight, and feel of it? If you can't jump in a nearby lake or ocean, try taking a soothing bath in Epsom salts.

Let your breath nourish your body. Stop, a few times each day, to take eight deep, mindful breaths. Inhale through your nose with the intent to fill your belly and then your lungs. Feel the breath as it slowly leaves your body through your mouth – releasing tension, troubles, and stress.

18. Embracing Your Spirit

There are so many things you can learn about, but
you'll miss the best things if you keep your eyes shut.
                                                        – Dr. Seuss

As important as it is to focus on our bodies, our diets, and removing stress from our lives, it is impossible to truly heal if we are lacking harmony with things greater than ourselves.

Let us now explore ways to become connected to our spirit.

Sacred Is the Space

My hope is that all of us could carve out a small area of our homes for a sacred space. This space may be as small as a prayer table, or as large as my "Zen" room.

I know I have joked about this room. In reality, it is the tiniest of the four bedrooms in our house – the one which served as a nursery when my children were young, and the first one to become empty as my children left the house. As soon as it no longer had an occupant assigned to it, I immediately grabbed it as my own and began sleeping in its twin bed on many a restless (and snoring) night. In it, and on its shelves, I have placed things which remind me of contemplation and meditation. When I enter it, it is a reminder to me to stop and think about what I am doing and where I am going. The space itself connects me to my spirituality.

I hope you can find a spot in your home to set up your own table; putting your personal beloved items in sight to use as a reminder for you to center yourself. These items can run the gambit from plants to pictures, beads to bibles, crystals to candles, flowers to "flotuses."

Walking in Circles

Have you ever taken part in a spiritual walk? One way to do so is to walk a labyrinth. If you are lucky enough to have a labyrinth at a local church, retreat house, or spiritual center, you should take advantage of it. There are labyrinths nearby at an arboretum and my local hospital as well.

People, formal cultures, and traditions have used the spiral and labyrinth designs as a symbol of their search for meaning and guidance. The labyrinth is non-denominational. Whatever one's religion (or lack of it) walking a labyrinth clears the mind and gives insight.

The moving meditation experienced in a labyrinth can be anything you wish it to be. The purpose is simply to walk with intent. Some people employ a mindful walking practice to just "be" with their bodies in the absence of judgment. Others use rosary beads or repetitive prayers. Still others use the same walk for a time of surrendering – a quieting of thoughts, worries, suffering, or grief. The center rosette should be used as a place of meditation; the outward walk back, a way of letting in good energy and thoughts.

Meditations regarding circles arise from the compelling need to know our own reality, to align this knowing with our body's wisdom, and to awaken in ourselves a sense of being in harmony with the universe. I'm sure we've all seen a drawing of circular designs called mandalas. The word "mandala," translates as "sacred circle." Hindus and Buddhists use them as a spiritual and ritual symbol, usually representing the cosmos or universe.

Circular forms abound in the natural world as well. In the circle there is no beginning and no end. The circle is eternal.

So, my friends, are we.

Buddhist Philosophy and Chronic Illness

The Dalai Lama has been quoted as saying, "Do not use Buddhism to become a Buddhist; use it to become better at whatever else in your life you are doing already."

While I had always envisioned myself a Buddhist wannabe (perhaps because we share a broad face and a round little belly) I admit I didn't know much about the actual practice of Buddhism, until I stumbled upon the book, *How to Be Sick: A Buddhist-Inspired Guide for the Chronically Ill and their Caregivers* by Toni Bernhard. As the Dalai Lama suggests, I have since found myself embracing these aspects of Buddhist philosophy and incorporating them into my fragile mindset in order to help me deal with my illness:

Suffering is present in the life of all people. We benefit from accepting the fact that all humans are subject to change and disease. It happens differently for each person. I need to accept that this is the way it is happening to me. Now. At this present moment.

Life is susceptible to impermanence, change, uncertainty, and unpredictability. Although we yearn for just the opposite, we need to accept the fact that life circumstances, like the weather, will blow us from here to there from time to time.

There is no fixed or unchanging self. Although I may be dealing with illness inside my body, I am not a sick person.

I have also gained insights from reading other books about Buddhist philosophy (confession: *Buddhism for Dummies*.) I recognize the fact that many of these insights are simply different ways of stating the same values taught in my own Christian faith, yet Buddhist teachings are nearly always neatly tucked into nice lists for me to remember. The Buddha's eightfold path to the secession of suffering could also be called, *A Guide to Right Living* and consists of the following:

Right View
Right Intention
Right Speech
Right Action
Right Livelihood
Right Effort
Right Mindfulness
Right Concentration

Buddhists and Hindus both believe that living a life consistent with these principles will stop the cycle of reincarnation, or "samsara" and allow your soul to be at rest in perfect peace, happiness, and emptiness. While I may not be striving to reach this state of Nirvana, I *am* striving for a way to accept my suffering so that it doesn't overtake my life; leaving me jealous, self-absorbed, and regretful. Bernhard's book offers the following techniques which I now try to practice in order to overcome the emotional toll which my illness has brought.

Cultivating Joy in the Joy of Others – This is an exercise to help get rid of that envy I feel when seeing others leading relatively normal and carefree lives. I *should* rejoice in the joy of others. Can you give me a reason – short of jealousy and selfishness – why I would I refrain?

Well Wishing towards Myself and Others – This is a practice (called Metta meditation) I can employ towards any individual in my life. I practice wishing them the very same things that I wish for myself. Even if wishing certain people well may seem hard or insincere at times, it is the Buddhist way of praying for all those around me and reminding me to greet everyone in my life with friendliness and loving kindness.

Using Compassion to Alleviate Suffering – In a way, we have already covered this in the tai chi section of this book. This technique makes us grateful towards our bodies and all they do for us each day.

Opening My Heart to the Suffering of Others – In order to take part in this, we are instructed to breathe in the suffering of others and breathe out measures of kindness, serenity, and compassion.

The truth is that nothing gives you a sense of humility, teaches you compassion, and enables you to order your priorities like an encounter with illness, grief, or sorrow.

Nothing.

If you, my friends, think yourself one of the fortunate ones who have not yet encountered any of the above, you might just take a moment to consider yourself among the unlucky – for you have not experienced the fullness of life which the cosmos has in store for you.

The Power of Prayer

I first intended to leave this section out of this book. Incredulously, my memoirs were going to tout the wisdom of Buddhist philosophy while leaving the comfort and curative power of my own Christian faith (along with the world's two other monotheistic religions) with only a passing mention. It was easy for me to embrace a quote from the Dalai Lama and cherry-pick through Buddhist practices, but it took a bit more delving to understand the Christian doctrine on suffering. (Perhaps I needed *Christianity for Dummies*???)

The debate about the role of prayer in healing has been active for decades. Some studies have shown that distant or intercessory prayer has improved healing in patients who were not even aware they were being prayed for. It has also been proven that the very act of praying evokes a relaxation response which, like meditation, quells stress, quiets the body, and promotes healing. Almost all religions employ some sort of prayer beads in order to recite repetitive prayers or devotions. These beads tend to order the pace of an individual's breathing; inviting them to become calm and serene.

But this is not the power I want to explore in this section.

I am sure that each individual faced with acute or chronic illness at one time or another wrestles with the question, "Is there a reason for my suffering?" or "Why do bad things like this happen to good people?"

Buddhism and Hinduism are not the only two religions which wrestle with this concept of suffering. The world's monotheistic religions, Christianity, Judaism, and Islam, all have their own outlooks on suffering. (Keep in mind that the term "suffering" is used here in a more traditional way than when we explored it in the context of Mindfulness or Buddhism.) While all three faiths view God as all-powerful, all-loving, and all-knowing, each deals with the concept of suffering in slightly different ways. The word, "Islam" itself means "submission." Many Muslims believe that suffering is allowed as a test of humility and faith. In this way, pain can lead to repentance and good deeds. Many Jews believe that we should not try to understand God's sense of justice, but because God suffers along with the sufferer, importance is placed on helping those who are suffering; the concept of "Tikkun Olam," or an act of kindness to repair the world.

Christians, too, acknowledge that suffering is an inescapable feature of human existence and every human person suffers in a variety of ways. Christianity's answer to the question of suffering is known as "Redemptive Suffering;" the belief that, like Christ's death on the cross, our own suffering can make an important good possible.

When he was pope, Benedict XVI said, "The cross reminds us

that there is no true love without suffering, there is no gift of life without pain." If I believe that salvation was brought about by Christ's suffering, then my suffering, too, can be transformative. Just like the Buddhist practice which was described as "Opening My Heart to the Suffering of Others," by uniting myself with the cross I should be able to embrace pain and change it into something beneficial.

I have learned that others can be helped as a result of my suffering. I have already written about how the timing of my own illness coincided with Leah's; leaving us both at home to help and support each other. It also arrived just in time to deal with my father's illness. I was able to spend the last nine months of my father's life helping my mother with her daily visits to the nursing home. I hope that the free time I gained by no longer working was put to use to help alleviate some discomfort for both of my parents.

I have yet to decide if I believe that suffering is randomly dispensed by an imperfect world, if it is simply the yin to happiness' yang, or if God's plan is minute enough to have assigned this to me. I do not need to know. Of all of the things in my life that are impossible to control, the one remaining thing which I do have power over is my reaction to life's circumstances.

And so I trust that my suffering will be beneficial. My illness has allowed me to gain strength through my weakness. It has expanded my world, drawn me closer to God, and allowed me to become more serene, humble, and compassionate. I have been lifted above my circumstances and am truly more alive now than I was when I appeared to be perfectly healthy.

19. Coping Mechanisms

I know it is wet and the sun is not sunny.
But we can have lots of good fun that is funny.
– Dr. Seuss

Fatigue Fighters

I am not sure that I have much to add on this topic but will try.

A Good Night's Sleep – I have found that those rare and precious nights when I experience a good night's sleep will provide a tremendous boost for me the next day. I know that I need much more sleep than the average person and aim for a minimum of ten hours each night. Keep in mind that many of these hours in bed are spent tossing, turning, sweating, sipping, and wall-hugging. My sleep is constantly being interrupted by physical discomfort and I never know when the dreaded insomnia is going to hit and leave me sleepless for hours on end.

Naps – Needed, Needed, NEEDED!

Exercise – As discussed earlier, conventional wisdom states that regular exercise will help fend off fatigue. I am not exactly sure that these experts have ever experienced the *Walking Dead Wipeout* after a mere block or two, but I can tell you that my tai chi classes energize me. It is up to you to figure out just what works for you and your body.

Pacing Activities – I find that this is hands-down the most important factor in warding off fatigue. As much as I might like to attempt to do on those days when I feel I have some energy to spare, I have learned that I need to pace myself. I am now an official one-stop shopper. And this works both ways. On days when I don't feel good, I try to force myself out of the house to run one errand, even if it is a trip to a drive-up ATM. On days when I feel better, I still limit myself to two errands; for if I don't I will quickly find I have blown it all.

Lightening the Load

It is hard for a control freak who is used to doing it all to find that she's experiencing trouble even doing some. In the past, I never liked sending another family member to the grocery store because I didn't think they would purchase exactly the items I would have chosen. I planned every dinner, cooked every meal, did the dishes, paid the bills, prepared the taxes, took the animals to the vet, and lugged the dog food home from the store – all with a 50 hour work week.

That mindset is a thing of the past. I now take help anywhere and everywhere I can get it.

Online shopping has become my best friend. I use at-home delivery for my big grocery, toiletries, and cleaning supply purchases – freeing me up to go to smaller markets for meats and produce. I am a prime member at a major online retailer and have found that I can order anything from coffee, to candles, to curtains and have them delivered in two days. I routinely order a 26 pound bag of dog food to be delivered without shipping charges in a mere three days.

My husband has certainly picked up much of the slack, cooking and shopping more than he ever used to. And, even though I'm no longer working, I still have a cleaning service come to the house every other week.

Lucky, I know.

Comic Relief

In order to navigate through the physical and emotional maze of chronic illness, the more imaginative among us will find themselves fine-tuning their coping skills by inviting humor into the equation. I can only envision that these mechanisms vary widely from person to person. You, my friends, will now be fortunate enough to hear mine.

Despite the fact that I carried my immune-challenged daughters in my womb for a long eight months prior to their premature births and subsequently nursed, fed, and laundered their thongs for countless years afterwards, I find that they seem to be quickly tiring of my complaints. I ask you, who do you think it was that rejoiced in their very first steps? Why then, should they roll their eyes if I utter a small "ouch" as I slowly walk through a room?

And do those children think they were born into the Flying Walenda Family? If not, why do they think there is something wrong as the woman who held her breath in fear as she taught them to how to navigate a set of stairs winces a little as she tries to descend those very same obstacles?

So I am relegated to the role of suffering servant. In case you didn't know, the suffering servant is always silent. And so I invented a game which allows me to bear my pain in noiseless agony while remembering to be thankful. I call it the, *"Things Could Always Be Worse"* game. This is a diversion wherein I imagine the worst possible scenario for each and every pain I encounter:

> **Example 1:** When my toes or feet hurt I tell myself, "There are people who have had their feet crushed in automobile accidents. Thank God I don't have to deal with that!"

> **Example 2:** As I convulse with my ubiquitous morning cough, I think about those with chronic lung disease and know that it could be worse.

And so I pass my time envisioning a host of those worse off than I am: tuberculosis and ebola patients, paraplegics, denture wearers, accident and burn victims, comatose individuals, those with kidney stones, alopecia, leprosy, or congestive heart failure, as well as those unfortunate individuals with frontal lobe lobotomies.

I invite you to try this with me just one time to see how it feels. Imagine yourself in the shower one morning, cursing the fact that you have to bend over to shave your legs because the particular up and down motion associated with shaving tends to sever your life energy from you. Now imagine yourself thinking, "There are people in full body casts who are not able to bend over at all" or – better yet – "There are people who, through some accident of nature, are incapable of growing hair."

Putting aside the fact that some reader out there is now

imagining the poor soul who cannot produce enough tears to have a good cry or sufficient saliva with which to swallow food, don't you suddenly feel better about your own ailments?

Another game I employ is one based on a Buddhist practice covered in Toni Bernhard's book, *How to Be Sick*, but my warped-yet-witty mind has adapted the practice for my own comic use.

It just so happens that the name of the mindfulness practice which Bernhard calls *Drop It* already had a humorous connotation in our household. When our dog Kasey was a puppy we employed the command called *Drop It* which was intended to stop that retriever from putting unwanted things in her mouth. If she picked up a wayward sock or unattended sticky boob and stored it in her mouth, the command would make the item magically cascade from her mouth as she ran over to the treat jar to get her reward.

One summer, years ago, Kaitlyn and my niece were walking the dog. My niece became enthralled with this particular command which was invariably put to the test on each walk, for there is always something fascinating and new to explore in the wide world of retrieverland. Wondering if it was just the tone used which produced such marvelous results, my niece then replaced the doggie command *Drop It* with the not-so-polite phrase, *Poop on Your Head*. Sure enough, *Poop on Your Head*, when emitted in the same authoritative tone, produced identical results and – from that moment forward – *Poop on Your Head* became a favorite idiom in our household.

In reality, the Buddhist-inspired practice of *Drop It* is not far removed from the idea behind the dog command. Just like it is not productive for your average retriever to secrete a sock in the recesses of her mouth, neither should we be hosting negative thoughts. It is only when these thoughts are brought to the forefront that we can acknowledge them for what they are and then carefully dismiss them.

So you can imagine that when I first attempted to practice *Drop It*, my mind got rid of the negative thoughts it needed to, by replacing it instead with doggie droppings. At first I was dismayed to find my disturbed mind wandering to such base levels, but eventually I accepted it for what it truly was – a way to put things into perspective and make me chuckle; for "poop" is really the essence behind those negative feelings.

Yet I would be lying if I left you with the impression that cleansing my mind of negative beliefs is the only way I employ the *Poop on Your Head* idiom. I know I told you earlier that I spend time each morning wishing good things to those around me but sometimes – just sometimes – I secretly find myself wishing that doggie dropping phrase on other people as well.

As you can see, I still have a little work to do on my inner self.

Part Four: On the Outside Looking In

20. The Doctor/Patient Fit

When at last we are sure you've been properly pilled,
then a few paper forms must be properly filled,
so that you and your heirs may be properly billed.
— *Dr. Seuss*

While navigating through my family's various illnesses I have had the opportunity to interact with a number of physicians. Because lupus and Sjogren's are systemic diseases, affecting many different organs or systems in your body, those who suffer from these disorders need to see a number of specialists to deal with different aspects of their disease.

While a rheumatologist manages my overall care and deals with my complaints of joint and muscle pain, she does not have the expertise to deal with all of the complications which come with the disease. I currently see an optometrist and cornea specialist for my eye health; a neurologist for peripheral neuropathy; a gastroenterologist for GERD, swallowing, and gastritis issues; a hematologist to monitor my antibodies and infusions; a dermatologist to deal with skin rashes and sun sensitivity; and a podiatrist to help determine what the heck has caused my toes to go all akimbo on me.

Yet, I am convinced that Leah holds the world's record for physician visits as she has dealt with Guillain-Barre and its aftermath. In addition to her general practitioner and rheumatologist, she has been seen by four different neurologists, a neurosurgeon, urologist, gynecologist, uro/gynecologist, optometrist, ophthalmologist, two endocrinologists, an infectious disease doctor, dermatologist, immunologist, two gastroenterologists, a pulmonologist, a pain management specialist, and an integrative medicine practitioner.

I wish I could offer you a surefire way to find just the right doctor – one who is knowledgeable, compassionate, collaborative, and holistic in nature. I recognize the fact that the process should be better than trial and error and so I try to obtain recommendations from other physicians or fellow patients, but that has not always worked as I would hope. Because our ailments are certainly not run-of-the-mill illnesses, I admit that I have sometimes been a bit of a credential snob – researching a physician's schooling, residencies, and fellowships – but have also found that those trained or practicing at top-notch hospitals do not always have the time or interest in dealing with those who are not on their deathbed.

A 2014 American Autoimmune Related Diseases Association survey revealed that, on average, it takes four years and five different physicians for a patient to receive an accurate diagnosis. In addition, the survey revealed that 13 percent of the physician respondents received no autoimmune disease education at all and only 22 percent received five or more lectures. Half of the physicians who responded stated that they were uncomfortable with diagnosing autoimmune diseases.

Although I am the type of individual who never wants to make waves or – God forbid – have others think I don't like them, I have found that this philosophy does not work when dealing with chronic illness. Waiting in timid anticipation for return phone calls and test results is agonizing. Taking a physician's diagnosis (or lack of one) at face value when it doesn't seem right in your gut, is counterproductive. Second opinions are critical when you sense that your symptoms have been dismissed or a diagnosis is not correct. Just use Leah's diagnostic tangle as an example. How many times have we all heard that you have to be your own advocate when dealing with your health? How true it is!

Becoming your own advocate has its responsibilities. In order to hold up your end of the bargain, you need to learn about autoimmunity, your disease, and your doctor. I have also learned the hard way that you need to become familiar with the side effects of medicines prescribed. Yes, some of these diseases and medications are complicated, but isn't it worth your time to understand what is going on inside your own body? Would you go into battle without sizing up your opponent's strength?

One of the cardinal rules of advocacy is this: Know thy blood! Of course, I have had many years of practice. I quickly discovered the value in learning how to read the results of my daughters' extensive blood tests, along with their other diagnostic testing. I needed to understand their respective diseases in order to try to make sense of what was happening to my family. I could not sit with one of the preeminent pediatric rheumatologists in the world every six weeks and not want to be informed. And as is true with all things, knowledge is power. I have found that the best doctors are the ones who work collaboratively with their patients.

I have also come to the conclusion that – especially in the murky waters of some specialties – all physicians do not think and label alike; nor do they necessarily speak the same language. One rheumatologist may call a condition "like" lupus, while another may call it undifferentiated connective tissue disease. Are they the same thing? One endocrinologist may not treat an elevated TSH (indicating possible thyroid problems) and wait until a patient's T3 or T4 are found to be out of whack, but another will. An integrative practitioner (who just might stay away from labels) may treat her patients with dried pig's thyroid, while another endocrinologist will treat with a synthetic hormone.

I recently attended a medical school graduation where the newly-named doctors swore what used to be referred to as a "Hippocratic Oath." In it were several passages which made me stop and think. I was particularly struck by these two:

> **That I will** recognize the limits of my knowledge and pursue lifelong learning to better care for the sick and to prevent illness.

> **That I will** seek the counsel of others when they are more expert so as to fulfill my obligation to those who are entrusted to my care.

I am convinced that all physicians enter the medical field with the most noble of intents. They all share the desire to help others. I realize that some are smarter, or better trained, than some of their peers. I am only asking for attention, knowledge and, yes, some research if the symptoms I am presenting are of a nature you have not dealt with since clinical rotations in medical school. I am also asking you to recognize the limits of your experience and respect my right to get a second, or more specialized, opinion.

Imagine my dismay when, after waiting three months for an appointment, the first neurologist I visited told me that Sjogren's only causes large fiber neuropathy. Once he performed a nerve conduction study and found no abnormalities in my large fiber nerves he erroneously proclaimed that the loss of feeling in my feet and legs was coming from a pinched nerve in my back. Now, readers, even

YOU know that Sjogren's can (and does) cause small fiber neuropathy. I tried my best to debunk his diagnosis, telling him what I had read and where I had read it, but still he stood firm. The entire encounter was a loss for me – a loss of precious time, resources, and confidence in the medical profession.

While the next neurologist agreed that Sjogren's can cause small fiber neuropathy, he would not definitively diagnose me with it because he thought it didn't really matter. It does – on so many levels. Not only do I want to know what is happening to my body for my own peace of mind, I need to know for the future of my daughters. Let me also tell you that putting a "most likely" in front of a diagnosis does not cut it when applying for disability. This very same physician, when I brought back the findings and recommendations from the Sjogren's specialists, refused to take them for my file and would not prescribe the IvIG infusions I needed. I wanted to bring that Hippocratic Oath to him and shove it in his face.

Bear with me while I offer a sampling of just a few more physicians who may have run awry of their original intent and should send you running as well:

The Fast Talking Physician – This is the guy who races through medical terminology like a desperate bachelor on a speed date. Slow down please! Did you not order that MRI of my brain because I admitted to you that I suffered from drain clog?

The Do-Nothing Doctor – This one spies the vast array of specialized tests already performed and so opts to run a simple CBC and metabolic panel just to make you think she's doing something. Oh yes, and she may listen to your heart with a stethoscope because insurance companies pay doctors to do that sort of thing.

The Intimidating Internist – This is the one who, when you call to tell them that a certain medication does not seem to be as effective as it once was, boldly asks you, "Well why not?" Who's the doctor here????

The "Oh My" Orthopedist – This is the foot and ankle specialist who – when trying to roll my ankle about – declared, "Your ankle is so stiff!" Welcome to the amazing world of arthritis. Just because I didn't injure my foot while training for a marathon doesn't mean it isn't painful.

The Ophthalmologist Who Doesn't Look – Can you at least glance at my chart before you start speaking to me about my aging eyes??? I shouldn't have to remind you that there's a completely different reason why my eyes don't produce the tears they used to.

The Mispronouncing Medic – I immediately lose confidence in any physician who mispronounces Sjogren's (show-grins) or Guillain-Barre (ghee-yan bhay-ray) Syndromes.

The Portal Practitioner – I'm all for simplifying communication, but don't send a cryptic message via your patient portal to my daughter who has just communicated to you that her symptoms are getting worse by the hour, simply stating, "Nothing of significance" or very soon we will be discussing another portal even though you're not a proctologist.

The Egregious Employer – This is the physician who allows Nefarious Nurses, Paperwork Pirates, and Front Desk Forsakers all to be part of the office staff. Patient interaction is important on all levels.

Although I may make it sound like the ideal doctor is of the same ilk as Santa Claus and the Easter Bunny, I have indeed encountered competent and compassionate physicians. I have sat with my daughters' rheumatologist for a full hour as we worked through Leah's symptoms and findings.

My own rheumatologist is knowledgeable and conversant in the many pitfalls of Sjogren's Syndrome. She recognizes the fact that the accompanying fatigue and joint pain can be disabling and is supportive of my decision to leave work. She has also been very supportive of my decision to seek treatment at the Sjogren's Center and has taken their expert advice regarding my care. And of course, I am overwhelmed and comforted by the competence of the rheumatologist/neurologist who now oversees my care there. He not only understands the many and varied manifestations of this disease I live with, he is actively working to find better treatments through his research.

Just think about that oath again for a minute. The second clause ends with, ". . . my obligation to those who are entrusted to my care." I have entrusted myself to these physicians' care and, in turn, I need them to simply have a big heart, a working brain, and a modest ego which will allow for a collaborative spirit.

As Dr. Seuss might phrase it, the rest will most indubitably follow.

21. The "Haves" and "Have Nots"

Now the Star-Belly Sneetches had bellies with stars.
The Plain-Belly Sneetches had none upon thars.
– Dr. Seuss

While we may have exhausted the topic of my family's illnesses, we have not had the chance to speak about the ways in which chronic illness affects the loved ones of those burdened by disease. In my particular case this means my husband.

Alone.

Over the years I have sometimes felt sorry for surrounding Michael with an all-female family; excluding him from conversations based on boys and bras, blush and bronzers. Many was the time that one of them would tentatively traipse downstairs sporting two different shoes, asking for opinions on which one looked better with a particular outfit. Of course if I declared a winner, the losing shoe was automatically chosen. But it always made me chuckle to see Michael enter the discussion. Why in heaven's name did that man think that his engineering degree qualified him to enter the world of teenage fashion? Did that colossal brain of his not understand that it was put on this planet simply to fix their laptops, cell phones, and iPods?

These days I wonder just what it is like for Michael to be the sole survivor in a family filled with illness. Does he feel lucky? Lonely? Labored? Could it be that he feels that he has been cheated out of living a life he could have enjoyed more? Do you think that sometimes, late at night, he just might feel as if he had the misfortune to pronounce those wedding vows before the wrong woman 30 years ago? How would it feel to have an entire family counting on you to be the strongman? The sole breadwinner? The one expected to bear it all? I cannot quite call Michael my caregiver but yet he cooks more meals, does more shopping, and foregoes more fun than he ever did before.

How exactly does it feel to come home after working a ten hour day at a stressful job only to find your wife waking up from a three hour nap? Which wedding vow would prepare you for *that* emotion? And then there is the constant litany of complaints with which to contend. I'm sure it makes him think twice about leading off the dinner conversation with, "So how was your day, Honey?" Even I would encourage him to avoid falling into that trap.

And what about the "dump" texts? Michael has been the recipient of countless texts from me like: "I should never have come here, I don't even have the strength to drive home!" "My joints are killing me!" "Remind me never to try shopping again!" "You're on your own for dinner, Buddy, I'll be in bed!" Somehow, as the "dumper", I feel enormously relieved after unloading my grievances in a text. But I know that the "dumpee" doesn't feel better at all.

I also know from my own experience prior to joining my daughters' sorority, that living with, and loving, others with chronic illness can be heartbreaking, especially when those who are ill are your own children. Watching a spouse deal with a life-changing illness must be equally painful.

The needs of the "Have Nots" are often overlooked. They,

too, deal with worry, uncertainty, and the disquiet that comes about from shifting relationships. Many families also suffer from additional financial burdens brought about by the cost of health care, prescription drugs, over-the-counter remedies, complementary treatments, and reduction in income that chronic illness can bring.

It is estimated that 75 percent of marriages where chronic illness is present end in divorce. Even when compared to the generally agreed-upon notion that roughly 50 percent of all marriages end the same way, this statistic is still scary. A study of older couples at the University of Michigan found that risk of separation is higher when the wife, not her husband, was ill. Although this study focused only on cancer, heart disease, lung disease, and stroke, I can only imagine that these numbers would be higher when applied to autoimmune disease since autoimmunity affects women more often than men. Indeed, 78 percent of autoimmune sufferers are women. Add to this the fact that autoimmune diseases are sometimes impossible for others to understand fully, and I can only imagine that the risk of separation would be higher still.

I hope I have made it clear that this book is solely about my experiences, not those of my husband. This is only fair, for I would never want Michael to try to convey my emotions and feelings in some other forum. And so the response to my questions about how it feels to be a "have not" must remain unanswered, yet we – the "haves" – must remain committed to considering their needs. Those of us who are lucky enough to have others who support us should never take that for granted.

22. Search for a Cure

Unless someone like you cares a whole awful lot,
nothing is going to get better. It's not.

– Dr. Seuss

I hope that I have conveyed to you the very important reality that, without a cure for autoimmunity itself, there is absolutely no chance that I will breathe a sigh of relief. Even if pharmaceutical companies develop the correct drugs to somehow relieve each of my disparate symptoms, I will not be cured or whole again.

What about my daughters? Future grandchildren?

In many ways, the search for a cure is a game of numbers. Autoimmune diseases are the third most common category of disease in the United States after cancer and cardiovascular disease. In fiscal year 2015 the United States Office of Budget and Finance appropriated 4.9 billion dollars to the National Cancer Institute. Research on Heart Disease was awarded 1.3 billion. Autoimmune Diseases were appropriated just 821 million dollars.

The National Cancer Institute reports that there are over 14 million people living with cancer in the United States. The CDC estimates that 27.6 million Americans have been diagnosed with heart disease. And while estimates vary greatly between organizations, the conservative NIH estimate states that up to 23.5 million American suffer from autoimmune diseases. This means that the funds allocated for disease research by the United States government shake out like this: $350 per person for those living with cancer, $47 for each person with heart disease, and – at most – $35 per person for those suffering from all autoimmune conditions combined. What's more, autoimmune research is generally disease-specific and limited in scope.

The National Cancer Institute also receives private contributions through their Gift Fund, and we know that millions are donated to both the American Cancer Society and the American Heart Association. When was the last time you donated to one of the organizations which encompass the world of autoimmunity?

It is painfully clear that both public policy and private mindsets need to change if we are to find a cure for autoimmune diseases. We also need new drugs in the pharmaceutical pipelines; therapeutics that treat the entire disease, not just its symptoms.

Why the disparity?

Could it be due to the fact that the wide range of autoimmune diseases is not lumped together in one terrifying word like "cancer"? I believe that researchers now know that all cancers are not equal. Although the underlying process is always the same, different cancers attack the body in different ways and therefore require different treatments and protocols; so, too, autoimmune diseases.

And although autoimmunity does not cause death at the same rate as heart disease, autoimmunity can, in fact, kill both by direct cause (i.e. an adrenal crisis, pulmonary embolism, or stroke) as well as through complications encountered with a lifetime of living with the debilitating effects of a chronic disease.

Now for the confession of which I am not proud.

I bowed out of a study at the National Institutes of Health. I firmly believe that this study called, "The Pathogenesis of Sjogren's Syndrome" will prove to be useful to researchers who are attempting to tackle this disease.

As my first study date approached, apprehension and anxiety began to take center stage. Because it is not a cancer study, each participant must pay their expenses out of their own pocket. How could I, who was no longer working, justify the expense of the trip to begin with? Familiar worries and qualms then set in. How would I get to my appointment in the first place? Even if Michael worked it into a business trip and placed me on a shuttle to the campus, how would I navigate around it once I arrived? I attentively studied maps of the campus and the circuitous bus system within and saw no clear-cut answers. The literature referred to a free lunch. Where would that lunch be? What would I do as I ate by myself? Appointments were scheduled for me with a rheumatologist, dentist, and neurologist. Would I know how to navigate from one office to another? Was I pre-destined to experience the *Walking Dead Wipeout*? Believe me when I tell you that there are no words to describe what a mind in fear will begin to envision – and this was regarding my first appointment of many. In a moment of panic, I called and canceled my participation in the study.

And have felt a sense of shame ever since.

The gracious woman at the NIH told me that enrollment will continue to be open for a few years as they gather and confirm study participants.

How can I expect a cure – for both myself and my daughters – if I don't participate in helping to understand the root cause of the disease? And finding the root cause of this disease can only help in detecting the very essence of autoimmunity, would it not?

23. Showing Support

I meant what I said and I said what I meant.
An elephant's faithful one hundred percent.
– Dr. Seuss

Would you like to become a better spouse, sibling, child, or friend to those who are living with an autoimmune disease or other illness? Many people simply do not know where to start, uncertain of what to say or how to broach the subject. Although you have heard my story, I still think it helpful to share the following pointers:

Become informed about autoimmune diseases and conditions. It is hard to feel supported by someone who hasn't taken the time to become knowledgeable about our diseases and the process we battle.

Offer to accompany us to doctor or testing appointments. It is always nice to have a second set of ears to help remember what is discussed at these appointments – especially if one happens to encounter a *Fast Talking Physician*.

Help to lighten the load. Nearly everyone who suffers from autoimmunity experiences some level of fatigue and can only benefit by offers of help from others.

Try not to become judgmental. My symptoms may seem strange to you, but try not to apply your own perceptions to my experience. Take me at my word. No one can truly understand some of these symptoms without experiencing them firsthand.

Become a sounding board. When we talk, just listen. Sometimes we want advice and other times we just want to share our story.

Ask us how we feel. I cannot imagine anyone complaining about someone who asks too often, but have personally suffered heartache from those who never ask.

Let us know that we have not been forgotten. A note, email, call, or visit will help to reduce the sense of isolation.

Never underestimate the healing power of touch.

And finally,

Keep us real. Remind us that life is not all about us all of the time. We are responsible for caring for you as well. Tell us honestly if we are becoming self-centered and self-absorbed. It is easy to become enveloped in a disease and sometimes we need to be pulled out.

Part Five: Looking Forward

24. The Future for My Daughters

You're on your own
and you know what you know,
and YOU are the one who'll decide where to go.
　　　　　　　　　　　　　　　　　– Dr. Seuss

Last September we arrived at an important juncture in the life of my family, as all three of our daughters embarked on (or re-boarded) their paths to the future.

After time working in New York City as a media planner, Kaitlyn decided to become a physician. Almost five years after receiving a B.A. in English, she returned to school to take those numerous science and math classes that are prerequisites for entering medical school. Two years later Kaitlyn took her MCAT and began the application process. The holistic and hands-on approach to patient care practiced by osteopathic physicians resonates with her personal philosophy regarding health and wellness and so she is pursuing a degree as a Doctor of Osteopathic Medicine.

Of course Kaitlyn had flown from our nest years before, but it was a particular joy to see our happy-go-lucky-breach-born-baby move on to medical school. And while I do not often brim with anything these days, I was indeed brimming with pride as I sat next to Michael and watched the dean of the school place her medical coat on her at a white coat ceremony.

Why is it that our eldest has decided to become a physician?

Is it her nature? Her indomitable optimism? Or has her own encounters with illness – or those of her family – spurred her on? Kaitlyn has a big heart and the greatest sense of optimism I have ever encountered. She is sure to become a knowledgeable, collaborative, and compassionate physician.

Megan also decided to return to academia in order to attain her Masters degree in School Psychology. She moved to New York state to attend a three year graduate program with a two mile commute from a one bedroom apartment in a city where she didn't know a soul. Megan's time spent working as a vision therapist after getting her B.S. in Psychology served to pique her interest in the challenges associated with childhood learning and she would like to be part of the solution to the problem.

And Leah? Somehow, in the midst of all her ailments, something happened. Leah symptoms began to ease and she started to feel somewhat better. Her thyroid medicine was adjusted, and – although those hormones are not yet at optimum levels – she has felt improvement. She began to receive weekly, and then monthly, vitamin B12 shots. She was also placed on the anti-malarial medication that her siblings and I are already taking.

Is this improvement the result of any one specific thing? The cumulative effect of all three? Or are the residuals of Guillain-Barre Syndrome slowly coming to an end?

After more than two long and agonizing years spent largely on our family room couch, Leah spent the summer working as a hostess at a busy local restaurant, spending hours on her feet. Yes, it was hard on her body but she was determined to make it work. Success has built upon success and then, after an absence of two-and-a-half years, she returned to Delaware to finish the few remaining classes she needed to complete her undergraduate degree.

A nightmare over? Certainly not yet. There is still concern about many of her neurological and muscular issues, but we will take any relief we can get. Let's remember Leah's ill-fated Froggy ride, her dozens of dance trophies in basement boxes, the extraordinary Easter Egg cache accumulated by the child in the chiffon bathrobe.

Leah has what it takes. Let's just hope that fate restores it to her.

25.   And Me?

*Sometimes the questions are complicated
and the answers are simple.*

– Dr. Seuss

Because I have applied for Social Security benefits, I have recently received a third party questionnaire regarding my lifestyle.   In it, the SSA wants Michael to document just how my life has changed since the onset of my disability.   In the spirit of free disclosure I thought I would share just a few of his answers here:

Question: *Describe what the individual does from the time she wakes up until she goes to bed.*

Answer: *Enclosed please find a picture of a corner of our living room couch.*

Question: *What was she able to do before her illness that she can't do now?*

Answer: *Live like a normal human being.*

Question: *Does the illness affect her sleep?*

Answer: *Unlike Goldilocks, she is no longer able to find a bed, room, or sleep position that is just right.   On the bright side, she hasn't had the pleasure of being woken up by three bears staring at her either.*

Question: *Does the disabled individual do any shopping, and if so, how does she shop?*

Answer: Well for starters, let's just say that she will never again hear the words "Attention K-mart (or Walmart, Target, or Costco) Shoppers." If she can't buy it online, we don't have it in our house.

Question: How far can she walk before needing to stop and take a rest?

Answer: The exact distance from the front door of the pharmacy to the rear of the store where those who are sick are forced to trudge to pick up their prescriptions.

Question: If she has to rest, how long before she can resume walking?

Answer: However long it is until the person she has asked to save her place on the prescription line while she sits to rest indicates that it's her turn at the counter.

Question: Does she cook for herself or others in your family?

Answer: Well let's just say that she is able to prepare a lot of prepared foods.

Question: Have you noticed any unusual behavior in the individual since her illness began?

Answer: Would you view hugging a cold bedroom wall in the middle of the night as unusual?

Question: If there's anything else, please describe in your own words how this illness has affected the disabled individual.

Answer: The woman I live with now is not the woman I married. She has dried up before my eyes. She can no longer walk the dog, clean the house, cook her family dinner, or attend social events *without being assured a seat within five minutes of arrival. She sleeps slathered in battle gear with a humidifier at her side. I have held my breath numerous times as she has nearly choked while attempting to swallow simple foods. My ears are filled with her groans as she goes up and down stairs in our home. I sense a loss of confidence in her demeanor and a dread of facing others. I have watched as she has struggled to find words and felt her embarrassment when coming up empty-handed. Yes, I made a vow to be true to her in sickness and in health but right now I'm worried about what the future will bring.*

The perceptive souls among you may have already guessed that my husband didn't exactly pen those snarky phrases when he returned his questionnaire, but I believe he should have.

And that last answer about the woman he married? Those words, my friends, reveal my very real fears about what the future will hold for me. Without a cure, without a breakthrough, and without substantial relief from my symptoms, I fear that there is nowhere to go from here. I worry that, what might be a normal aging process for some, will be disastrous for me. What if I become even more affected than I am now? What if I acquire another autoimmune disease? And another? And, as we travel back to those wedding vows, I believe that Michael and I were as naïve regarding the "in sickness and in health" part as we were about what it was like to raise a family.

A few summers ago I witnessed a poignant moment between my parents, as my mother stood in my father's nursing home and fed him his lunch on their 64th wedding anniversary. Reminiscent of their wedding day when they each lovingly fed each other a forkful of wedding cake, I wondered what newlyweds in their right mind would ever envision the day when this feeding would become a necessity. And yet, my mother devotedly reenacted this scene day after day until my father could no longer eat.

I can't help but wonder: What will *my* movie look like before the final credits are played?

26. The Importance of Feathers

That one little feather she had as a starter.
But now that's enough, because now she is smarter.
— Dr. Seuss

I believe the time has come to wrap up this story, and it seems only fitting that we should close that woman's life-story right back in that movie theater where we started:

The film flashes forward to the following summer. A seagull caws from its perch on the neighbor's roof and the camera zooms in on our leading lady as she awakens in a sea green bedroom early one morning. Awkwardly cocooned in a bed sheet which tells the tale of one long and restless night, two wriggling feet are the only parts of her body that are visible. Very shortly we see an arm burst forth to rummage blindly around the nightstand for a vial of eye drops. Soon another is freed and the distinct sound of Velcro can be heard as one hand releases the other from their bondage in nighttime splints. Next, the rubber sleeping goggles are removed and those practiced hands guide the vial of drops carefully from one eye to the other. Aaaah! She sees sunlight reflecting off of the flamingo-hued house on the corner. That can only mean one thing.

This will be a morning worth getting out of bed for.

She emerges from that bedroom to find her husband and daughters, coffee cups in hand, attempting to plan the day's events. No matter how many times they have vacationed together in the family beach house, this morning meeting seems to be one they can't do without. Should they kayak? Rent paddleboards? Go to a winery? Brewery? That zoo they used to go to when they were little? She can see that Michael and Kaitlyn have already been on their morning run. The others, like she, still have the indistinct lines of pillows recently kissing their cheeks.

She doesn't listen to the plans others might make for the day; those plans are immaterial to her. There is only one item on our leading lady's agenda, and that item needs to be done before the sun travels much higher in the sky, so she slathers herself in sunscreen, grabs her speaker and chair, and turns her steps towards the beach.

"Wait!" her daughters call together. "We're coming with you!"

The mise-en-scene then changes to a gull's eye view of four females on an expansive beach at low tide. Spa music provides a sense of choreography as eight arms move together in measured unison. Yet soon we begin to hear a voice issuing instructions like, "Now pull the moon from the lake. . . receiving wisdom from the moon. Bring it up, share with the universe and release." It becomes apparent that our heroine is leading her daughters in a chi quong exercise, when the youngest daughter pulls a classic line out of the family annals and chirps, "This is re-dic-li-ous!" These three words bring back memories of the day the oldest endeavored to lead her sisters in a Native American rain dance. And, one by one, our quartet breaks into silly peals of laughter.

We next view our protagonist resting in her beach chair watching her daughters struggle to hold a one-footed pose while waves erode their tentative toehold in the sand. The echoes of little-girl squeals resound as she watches her medical school student, soon-to-be-psychologist, and recent college graduate begin to topple over, splashing each other with laughter as they do. Yes, she supposes it's true: If a man is as wise as a serpent, he can afford to be as harmless as a dove.

Knowing that her Zen moment has long passed, our heroine turns off the spa music and selects her "Psycho Sixties" playlist instead. A knowing audience can tell that our protagonist's sense of fancy is still at play when we hear her signature song:

> *She's come undun.*
> *She climbed a mountain that was far too high,*
> *and when she found out she couldn't fly,*
> *it was too laaaaate.*
> *She's come undun. . .*

Oh, how she loves to see her three daughters together! It doesn't happen often anymore, but she savors every moment when it does.

Empty nesters. That's what she and her husband are called now.

Of course they still have the pets – Kasey and Celiac Jax; the same cat with a new name. No surprise that the root of that cat's intestinal problems turned out to be autoimmune in nature. He found a home with the right family, that Jax did. Intolerance to grains is easy to handle in the feline world. And thank God that the cat's disease at least rhymed with his name. A rhyme is as good as an alliterative phrase to a poet.

Vegetarian dinners have flown out the window. Probiotics and biologics no longer reside in her refrigerator. Hair art is now a lost art in her home.

And the sixties beat goes on:

> *You don't know what we can find.*
> *Why don't you come with me, little girl,*
> *on a magic carpet ride. . .*

Her role of mother has undergone a transformation. She is no longer the matron of the Little House of Illness. Her daughters are not those who have been beaten by disease. She is, instead, the mother of three determined and optimistic young women who were willing to get off the couch and fly from that family tree in spite of the obstacles ingrained in it.

She is grateful that, whatever her failings as a mother, she never succeeded in holding her daughters back. She thinks about how much those three girls have taught each other about perseverance, confidence, and endurance; how much she, herself, has learned from them! And she can't help hoping that she just may have imparted some of the wisdom gained through her own experiences as well.

And then she hears it. Her heart flutters as she listens to the unmistakable crescendo of music preceding a song by Buffalo Springfield last heard in a movie theater all those months ago.

> *There you stood on the edge of your feather,*
> *expecting to fly.*
> *Well I laughed, I wondered whether,*
> *I could wave goodbye. . .*

I told you before that our heroine was not a brimmer, but something strange begins to happen to her eyes. She feels the familiar sensation associated with her body's impotent attempt at tear production, and suddenly her eyes brim over with unfamiliar moisture. That tightfisted tear sentry had been circumvented at last!

She sits back savoring those tears; envisioning each of her beautiful daughters poised on her own feather. Each feather a springboard to a promising future. Each future a bright star off in the distance.

But would their wings be unfettered?

Could they, indeed, take flight?

Helplessly hoping, she then raises those tear-filled eyes towards heaven and pleads, "Let them fly, dear Lord. Please help them fly!"

She then picks up her beach chair and turns her steps, and her pilgrim soul, towards home and her husband.

And that is the moment the closing credits begin to roll.

Closing Credits

American Autoimmune Related Diseases Association AARDA.org. *List of Diseases.*

American Autoimmune Related Diseases Association AARDA.org. *What Is the Family Connection in Autoimmune Diseases?*

Bernhard, Toni. *How to Be Sick.* Wisdom Publications, 2010.

Burmeister, Alice, and Tom Monte. *The Touch of Healing.* Bantam Books, 1997.

Donovan, Mary Ann, and Norman Latov. The Neuropathy Association. *A Guide to the Peripheral Neuropathies*

Donovan, Mary Ann, and Norman Latov. The Neuropathy Association. *Explaining Peripheral Neuropathy*

Faitweather, DeLisa; et al. The American Journal of Pathology. *Sex Differences in Autoimmune Disease from a Pathological Perspective* GBS-CIDP.org

GBS-CIDP.org

Karraker, Amerlia and Latham, Kenzie: Journal of Health and Social Behavior, In *Sickness and in Health? Physical Illness as a Risk Factor for Marital Dissolution in Later Life* September, 2015, 56 (3)

Keating, Thomas. *Open Mind, Open Heart.* 20th ed. Bloomsbury Academic, 2006.

Ladd, Virginia T., foreword, *As My Body Attacks Itself* by Dempewolf, Kelly Morgan, K2CS Books, 2014

Landlaw, Jonathan, et al. *Buddhism for Dummies.* 2nd ed. John Wiley and Sons, Inc., 2011

Lehman, Thomas J., M.D. *It's Not Just Growing Pains.* 1st ed. Oxford University Press, 2004

Lupus.org

The Moisture Seekers: Letter from Our CEO. Sjogren's Syndrome Foundation. Volume 34, Issue 7.

nccih.nih.gov. NIH National Center for Complementary and Integrative Health: *Acupuncture in Depth*

niddk.nih.gov. NIH National Institute of Diabetes and Digestive and Kidney Diseases: *Hashimoto's Disease*

nih.gov. US Department of Health and Human Services National Institutes of Health. *Estimate of Funding for Various Research, Condition, and Disease Categories.*

.

Rose, Noel. American Autoimmune Related Diseases Association AARDA.org. *The Common Thread.*

Sjogren's Syndrome Foundation. *The Sjogren's Book.* 4th ed., Oxford University Press, 2012

Wallace, Daniel J., M.D. *The Lupus Book.* Oxford University Press, 2000.

Wiesman, Janice F., M.D. *Peripheral Neuropathy.* Johns

Hopkins University Press. 2016.

Yeats, William Butler. "When You Are Old." *The Collected Poems of W. B. Yeats,* 2nd ed, edited by Richard J. Finneran, Simon and Schuster, Inc. 1989.

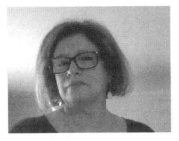

Meet the Author

Liz Wilkey is a graduate of Fairfield University and mother of three daughters with rheumatic and autoimmune conditions. Her unique life experiences, sense of humor, and appreciation of all-things-whimsical have combined to make her writing a joy to read. She currently resides in Morristown, N.J. with her dog, cat, and husband, Michael.

Q. Who are you favorite authors? I know it may sound cliché but I believe that Jane Austen and Charles Dickens would be the top two. I absolutely love their sense of humor along with their artful (and no-so-subtle) social commentary.

Q. What inspires you to get out of bed each day? I'll admit it's hard for someone like me to be "inspired" to get out of bed each day, but still I do. I have a very strong sense of responsibility and, in many respects, I feel the need to be "normal" and have an order to my day. Each morning I drink coffee, read the news, say prayers, and do other things that those who are not disabled do. Yes, sometimes I end up right back in that bed after two cups of coffee, but I attempt to get up each morning.

Q. Do you encounter obstacles while writing? Because Sjogren's Syndrome causes extreme fatigue, I am limited in the amount of time I can devote to writing each day. The dry eyes that Sjogren's brings also limits my time before a computer or tablet screen. And then there is the very-real problem of brain fog, where I cannot recall a word I need - much less know how to spell it. Writing and editing this book has been an slow process for me; an exercise in patience.

Q. What is you writing process?   With this book it was spontaneous. If not, it would not have the qualities of being cathartic and confessional. But really, it's all about revision. . .revision. . . revision. . .

Q. What is your e-reading device of choice? Because my autoimmune disease has caused me to have severe dry eye, I now do most of my reading through Audible. It is much more pleasurable for me to sit or lie with a warm compress on my eyes and listen, than to continue to injure and dry my eyes further by attempting to read - especially on an e-device or computer screen. And it turns out that I just may be an auditory, not visual, learner because I seem to absorb more of a book's content while listening. A big plus.

Q. Why the Dr. Seuss quotes? Seuss' book, *Horton Hatches the Egg,* was my hands-down favorite book when I was a child. I was also captivated with Stregna Nona and Emperor's New Clothes. I spoke earlier about my strong sense of responsibility and I believe these three books played a large part in forming my personality as an adult. I also resonate with Dr. Seuss' sense of whimsy, his optimism, intonation, and count. I have written many a child's poem in my day, and somehow they each end up sounding like a Dr. Seuss poem.